Nathan Bozeman

History of the Clamp Suture of the Late Dr. J. Marion Sims

and why it was abandoned by the profession

Nathan Bozeman

History of the Clamp Suture of the Late Dr. J. Marion Sims
and why it was abandoned by the profession

ISBN/EAN: 9783337881443

Printed in Europe, USA, Canada, Australia, Japan

Cover: Foto ©Andreas Hilbeck / pixelio.de

More available books at **www.hansebooks.com**

THE CLAMP SUTURE AND THE RANGE OF ITS APPLICABILITY, CONSIDERED IN RELATION TO THE CURE OF THE INJURIES INCIDENT TO PARTURITION, WITH STATISTICS.

BY NATHAN BOZEMAN, M. D.,

New York.

It was my intention in the outset to include in this paper a brief sketch of the early labors of every surgeon in the United States who had in any way contributed to the common fund of our knowledge relating to the injuries incident to parturition. But when the material accessible for the purpose had been collected, it was found that, to do justice to all, more space would be required than the limits of an article to be read before this society would warrant.

I have therefore restricted myself in the present consideration of the subject to the clamp-suture, as perfected in June, 1849,[1] by J. Marion Sims, M. D., then of Montgomery, Alabama, and what was accomplished with it by him and other surgeons in the United States and England (the only two countries in which it was ever used), outside of the Woman's Hospital of the State of New York. The cases treated by those surgeons constitute the first series. The cases treated individually by Dr. Sims in the Woman's Hospital by the same method form the second series.

The importance of the subject is sufficient to justify the

[1] *American Journal of the Medical Sciences*, January, 1852.

time and labor which I have bestowed upon it, and the statistics collected can not fail to prove of more than ordinary interest to the profession, in connection with the labors of Dr. Sims at this time, especially to the younger members of the society, who may not yet have a clear understanding of the peculiar difficulties that surrounded the treatment of the lesions in question only thirty years ago.

As one of the oldest if not the oldest operator now living in this country, I have to regret, as every one at all interested in the subject must, that Dr. Sims never published the statistics upon which rest his claims to priority of successful treatment of vesico-vaginal fistule. I always hoped that he would publish these statistics, knowing that they would place in a much clearer light the precise nature of the obstacles that he had to contend against in his early labors with the clamp-suture, and would at the same time prove interesting and profitable to the profession at large. Indeed, so thoroughly was I impressed with the importance of the subject, from all I knew about it from personal observation, and examination of the records of the Woman's Hospital, that, notwithstanding the differences of opinion between myself and Dr. Sims, as to certain claims of originality in the operation, which had existed for nearly a quarter of a century, I addressed him a letter in Paris urging the importance of his publishing these statistics, and promising him full co-operation in all that I could do in the way of assisting him. This letter, a copy of which is still in my possession, was sent to him through a friend in Paris March 19, 1879; but the inference is that he did not regard the matter of much importance, as the communication remained unanswered.

My reasons for addressing him upon the subject were fourfold: First, because we had been associated as partners years before, and had during that time treated jointly several most important cases of vesico-vaginal fistule with the clamp-suture, the complete details of which were in my possession; second, because the method of operating was peculiarly his own, and he had only the year before our association in practice published his account of it,[1] in which he made important claims of originality and success; third, because the method proved afterward defective in his own hands, especially in regard to urethro-vesico-vaginal and vesico-utero-vaginal fistules, which constitute more than one third of all the fistules met with in practice; and, fourth, because I had been one of the most strenuous advocates of the method, up to the time when I adopted the *new principles of gradual preparatory treatment and the button-suture.* Besides, having been charged by Dr. Sims with unfair criticisms upon his clamp-suture, I wished to modify these criticisms if he still thought they were, in any essential particular, unjust to him or to his claims.[2]

[1] *Loc. cit.*

[2] As it is not generally known by the profession precisely what relation existed between Dr. Sims and the writer at the period above referred to, and as great injustice has been done the latter by authors, both in this country and in Europe, growing out of the supposition that the relation was that of preceptor and student, which had been wantonly abused, with total disregard of honorable obligations and professional rights, it is proper to state in this connection the facts as they actually existed, since they form a part of the history of the subject under consideration, especially with regard to Dr. Sims's stand-point just after he had achieved his first complete success with his clamp-suture. The writer had previously been a private pupil and assistant of the late Dr. S. D. Gross (then Professor of Surgery in the University of Louisville, Ky.) for nearly three years, and had acquired from that eminent teacher a practical familiarity with surgical maladies generally, and with surgical methods of treating them. It was under these circumstances that he settled as a young practitioner in the city of Montgomery, Alabama, in June, 1849 (the same month that Dr. Sims states that he perfected his clamp-suture mode of operation), and was thrown in close relationship professionally with Dr. Sims. The result was that the writer was frequently called upon by him for assistance in his special operations for vesico-vaginal fistule, almost from their first acquaintance up to March, 1853, a period which included the date of Dr. Sims's first paper (January, 1852).

When Dr. Sims lost his health, from the combined ill effects of overwork and residence in the South, and was seriously entertaining the thought of removing with his family to a northern climate, he communicated to the writer his intention of settling in the city of New York, and asked him to purchase his house and lot in Montgomery. He urged as a reason that it was only by the sale of this property, for which there was little or no demand, that he could hope to carry out the necessary arrangements to enable him to make this proposed change of residence. The result was that the writer, on the ground of personal friendship, became the purchaser of his property on the terms that he

That there were real differences between Dr. Sims's ~~claims~~ and myself as to originality in the treatment of vesico-vaginal fistule, no better proof can be adduced than the publication of the statistics of the cases treated by our respective modes of operating, and the fact that he abandoned in the Woman's Hospital his original procedure,[1] only two or three weeks after the publication of my procedure.[2]

(Dr. Sims) proposed. In consideration of this favor, Dr. Sims associated himself with the writer in practice until the completion of his arrangements to leave the South for New York, which took place May 27, 1853, a little less than three months after this copartnership was formed.

In addition to these explanations, and in the same connection, the writer deems it important to state that Dr. Sims, soon after the dissolution of their copartnership, and when their differences with regard to certain claims of priority had sprung up, began to deny the originality of the labors of the writer in relation to his button-suture, and his modification of the lever-speculum, maintaining that this form of suture was no better than that of his clamp-suture, and at best could only be regarded as a slight modification of it, and of no practical value. As to the writer's modification of Dr. Sims's form of the lever-speculum, the latter objected to this as worse than useless. This he continued to do in various publications, not necessary to mention here (notwithstanding the fact of his early adoption of the writer's principle of gradual preparatory treatment, and his mode of adjusting interrupted silver sutures in the vagina), up to the time of his death, as shown by his autobiography, edited and published by his son within the last few months, entitled "The Story of My Life."

Here, on pages 316 and 364, are to be found references to the writer, together with his button-suture, and his modification of the lever-speculum, first used in a case by him in the service of M. Robert, at the Hôtel Dieu, Paris, November 16, 1858, and exhibited to Mr. Isaac Baker Brown and other surgeons in Europe, on other similar occasions, which not only are unjust to the writer, and disparaging in the highest degree to his legitimate claims of originality, but reflect seriously upon his honor.

It is true Dr. Sims is dead; but his words and sayings live, and enter into the literature of the subject under consideration, and deserve to be regarded as valuable, so far as they accord with principles and facts which are open to discussion by all. These will be presented for that purpose by the writer hereafter in a separate paper.

It is not the wish or intention of the writer in this communication to take notice of any disparaging reflections whatever, relating to his labors, by Dr. Sims, but simply to lay before the profession all the facts in detail appertaining to their respective claims of originality and priority, by which alone personal as well as scientific differences can be estimated and weighed.

[1] *Register of the Woman's Hospital of the State of New York from 1855 to 1862.*
[2] *Louisville Review*, May, 1856.

The important questions, therefore, presented for consideration are two: First, which of the two procedures, one with the *clamp-suture*, perfected by him June, 1849, *without gradual preparatory treatment*, and one with *gradual preparatory treatment and the button-suture*, perfected by me May 12, 1855, was best suited to the treatment of all classes of injuries incident to parturition? And, second, what was the range of applicability of each procedure, from the beginning of its adoption, as measured by the standard of success?

The peculiarities of the clamp-suture, first described by Dr. Sims, together with the principles upon which this form of suture was based, will now be presented, with the view of showing the range of its applicability, and the degree of success which attended its employment in actual practice.

Dr. Sims claimed for his procedure originality in these three particulars [1] (quoting from his first publication on the subject):

" 1. For the discovery of a method by which the vagina can be thoroughly explored, and the operation easily performed.

" 2. For the introduction of a new suture apparatus, which lies imbedded in the tissues for an indefinite period, without danger of cutting its way out, as do silk ligatures.

" 3. For the invention of a self-retaining catheter, which can be worn with the greatest comfort by the patient during the whole process of treatment."

" *Of the Position of the Patient for the Operation.*—With the exception of Velpeau and Chelius, all other operators, even Jobert, recommended that the patient be placed on the back, as in the operation of stone."

Dr. Sims *adopted* the teachings of the first two surgeons as to the advantages of the anterior positions, and selected as preferable for his purposes the *knee-elbow position.* His mode of exposing the fistule in this position was with what he called then " the lever-speculum," an instrument which had *long* been in use in Europe for the same purpose, but in which he made several important modifications and improve-

[1] *American Journal of the Medical Sciences*, January, 1852.

ments. In Dr. Sims's first employment of this position of the patient, and of this form of speculum, there is no doubt that his estimate of their value related almost exclusively to examinations of the vagina and uterus in their normal state. This is shown in the following quotations:

" An assistant on each side lays a hand in the fold between the gluteal muscles and the thigh, the ends of the fingers extending quite to the labia majora; then by simultaneously pulling the nates upward and outward, the os externum opens, the pelvic and abdominal viscera all gravitate toward the epigastric region, the atmosphere enters the vagina, and then, pressing with a weight of fourteen pounds to the square inch, soon stretches the canal out to its utmost limits, affording an easy view of the os tincæ, fistula, etc. To facilitate the exhibition of the parts, the assistant on the

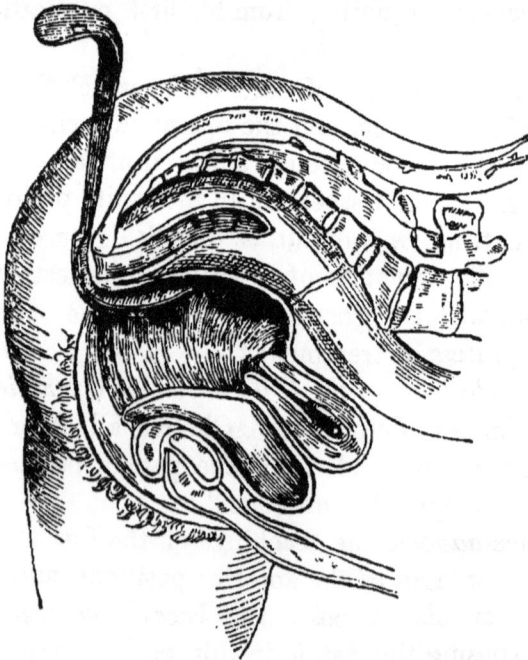

Fig. 1.

right side of the patient introduces into the vagina the *lever-speculum* represented in Fig. 1 [copied], and then, by lifting the perineum, stretching the sphincter, and raising up the recto-vaginal septum, it is as easy to view the whole vaginal canal as it is to examine the fauces, by turning a mouth widely open up to a strong light. This method of exhibiting the parts is not only useful in these cases, but in all affections of the os and cervix uteri requiring ocular inspection.

"The most painful organic diseases, such as corroding ulcer, carcinoma, etc., may be thus exposed without inflicting the least pain, while any local treatment may be instituted without danger of injuring the healthy structures. *By this method also a proper estimate, anatomically, can be had of the shape and capacity of the vagina ; for when there is no organic change, no contraction, and no rigidity of it from sloughs, ulcers, and cicatrices, and when the uterus is movable, this canal immediately swells out to an enormous extent, thus showing its great expansibility.*"

With regard to the suture apparatus perfected by Dr. Sims, as before stated, he says : "The one that I use for closing vesico-vaginal fistulæ I have termed the clamp-suture, from its peculiar method of action. Thus, if the profession allow me to introduce a new suture by its most appropriate name, we shall then have in general use sutures named, first, according to their relation, the interrupted and continued; second, according to the method of securing them, the quilled and twisted; and, third, according to its method of action, the clamp-suture. As all sutures are but modifications one of another, so is the clamp a modification of the quilled."

. . . .

(Fig. 2, copied, illustrates the apparatus applied to a vesico-vaginal fistule occupying the most favorable position for its use in the vesico-vaginal septum.)

"This suture is far preferable to anything before suggested for the purpose. Its introduction dates from June, 1849, since which time I have had comparatively little trouble in the treatment of the great majority of cases of vesico-vaginal fistula. Properly applied, *this suture never ulcerates out*, having always to be removed by means of scissors, hooks, and forceps. It may be allowed to remain intact for six, eight, or ten days, or even longer. If removed too soon, the delicate cicatrix may gradually yield to the traction of the ascending uterus, or to the force exerted by the bladder in expelling its contents, and reproduce a small fistulous orifice, to be closed by a subsequent and more cautious operation. I have seen the new cicatrix give way from another cause, and perhaps it is the chief one. *The clamps, burrowing in the vaginal surface, leave a deep sulcus or fissure on each side of the new cicatrix, which, when they are removed too soon, fill up by granulation. It is a law of all granulating wounds to contract as they heal, and this contraction on each side of the new cicatrix is often sufficient to pull it apart.* But if the clamps are allowed to remain till their sulci are covered with mucous membrane, then there is no danger of this accident, for these closures then gradually disappear, less by filling up with granulations than by an absorption of their elevated edges.

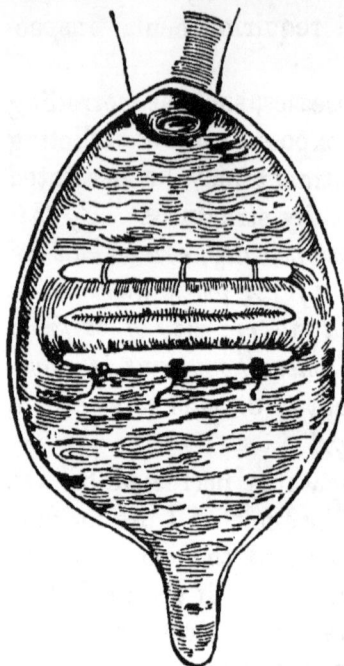

Fig. 2.

"Accidents of this sort have happened repeatedly in my hands, from a too early removal of the suture apparatus. Great judgment, which experience alone can give, is necessary to determine the length of time that the sutures ought to remain intact, for no positive rules can be laid down that will answer invariably in every case.

"I have also seen serious mischief result from leaving the clamps too long imbedded in the parts. *Then burrowing and ulceration may extend entirely through the vagino-vesical structure, thereby substituting new fistulous openings for the original one.* This complication is by no means incurable, but only prolongs the treatment and postpones ultimate success.

"In two or three instances I have witnessed a still more serious accident from an undue pressure of the clamps, viz., *a strangulation of the inclosed fistulous edges, which unfortunately resulted in a sloughing of the tumefied parts, and a consequent enlarging of the opening.* In no instance, however, has this accident rendered the case hopeless, or even caused me to feel any concern either for the immediate safety of the patient, or for ultimate success in treatment."

Next, with regard to the *modus operandi* of the self-retaining catheter proposed by Dr. Sims as an essential feature of his procedure. (See Fig. 3.) Of this he says : " *When*

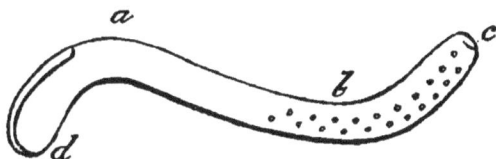

Fig. 3.

well fitted to the case, it can be worn with much ease to the patient, and never turns, never slips out, it matters not whether she lies on the back or side. It is perfectly self-retaining, being held in the bladder by an internal pressure against the symphysis pubis, and by external pressure on the outer end exerted by the labia overlapping it, and hiding it entirely from view." (Italics by the writer.)

In conclusion, Dr. Sims speaks of his labors in connection with his new operation, and of the circumstances under which he perfected it, together with his experience in its use, in these words :

"I have now completed what I have to say in a general way on the subject of the operation for vesico-vaginal fistula. It remains to detail individual cases, which will prove the curability of the disease, and also illustrate the varieties and complications to which it may be liable. The cases that occurred to me early, and which were given to me for the sake of experiment, will show the difficulties that had to be overcome, the many disappointments that had to be borne, and the ultimate success that crowned my efforts after the perfection of the mechanical contrivances, which, as it will be seen, was the work not of a day, and the result not of accident, but of long, laborious, and persevering application.

"But this communication has already reached to such an extent that I must postpone the relation of my cases to a future opportunity."

It is evident from all that Dr. Sims says in the extracts given above, from his first paper upon the subject of vesico-vaginal fistule, that he never entertained the idea of applying the clamp-suture to any other form of fistule than that of vesico-vaginal, involving the vesico-vaginal septum alone. Such a mechanism as that requiring the burrowing of the apparatus into the tissues, thereby becoming *concealed* from view, and having to be *searched* for in the tissues with a probe, when it did not occasion the more disastrous result of *strangulation and sloughing* of the borders of the fistule, can only be associated with the favoring conditions of a small fistula occupying a central position in the vesico-vaginal septum, and with those of a like size and position in the recto-vaginal septum.

The pressure necessary to bring about this peculiar mechanism of the clamps described, could not fail in any form of fistule involving the junction of the trigone of the bladder and the urethra, and attended with loss of tissue—designated as a urethro-vesico-vaginal fistule—to produce the gravest complications. In those forms involving the junction of the *bas-fond* of the bladder and the cervix uteri with loss of tissue—known as vesico-utero-vaginal fistules—the apparatus could only be applied, and that with the greatest difficulty, in a few exceptionally simple cases.

Dr. Sims's omission, in the preparation of his paper, to describe and illustrate these last two forms of fistule, as he did the one of vesico-vaginal fistule, is conclusive either that he had had no experience in their treatment at that time, or that he recognized the fact that the clamp-suture was not applicable to the management of such lesions — the more probable explanation. It is unfortunate that he did not record his early experience touching these important points, as it would have given the profession the practical data needed for a proper understanding of the subject. Some two years after this paper appeared, Dr. Sims published the details of four cases—three simple vesico-vaginal fistules and one vesico-utero-vaginal fistule; but this number was too small to be of any practical value in determining so important a question as the one whether his method, as described, was applicable to the treatment of the two classes of lesions referred to.

That Dr. Sims in his early experience had the opportunity of observing the lesion of urethro-vesico-vaginal fistule, as well as that of vesico-utero vaginal fistule, there can be no doubt. This opinion is based on the well-known fact that the proportion of the class of vesico-vaginal fistules, with which he was familiar, bears a more or less definite relation, not only to the class of vesico-utero-vaginal fistules (a case of which he reported, as stated), but to all other classes of fistules and injuries incident to parturition. Therefore it is reasonable to infer that his field of observation and study, when he wrote his paper on the application of the clamp-suture to the treatment of the simple class of vesico-vaginal fistules, was sufficiently wide to include as well the proportional numbers, at least, of the classes of urethro-vesico-vaginal and vesico-utero-vaginal fistules; and that his failure to point out their special treatment by his new mode of operating arose from a consciousness of the inapplicability of the method to these lesions, rather than from the want of opportunity for trial.

I would state here that my conclusions, with regard to the inapplicability of the clamp-suture to the successful treatment of urethro-vesico-vaginal fistules, were based on personal observations of some of Dr. Sims's own patients, during the early period of his employment of the method.

The same may be said to have been true of my conclusions as to the class of vesico-utero-vaginal fistules, though
the inapplicability of the apparatus here existed in a less
marked degree; there being a small proportion of these cases,
unattended with loss of tissue in the *bas-fond* of the bladder
and cervix uteri, that really could be cured with it by a judi-
cious adaptation.

I would also state, from my personal observation of Dr.
Sims's general practice with the clamp-suture, that it was
almost wholly inapplicable to that large proportion of cases
belonging to all the classes of fistules and injuries, urinary,
fecal, and perineal, complicated with plastic exudations about
the vagina and uterus, with cicatricial contractions, bands, and
bridles of the vagina, with immobility of the borders of the
co-existing fistule or fistules, and with fixation of the uterus.

It is a remarkable fact that Dr. Sims, in his first paper,
on the treatment of vesico-vaginal fistule, made no mention
of cicatricial contractions of the vagina as complications of
the affection, thus showing that he either regarded them as
insurmountable by any sort of treatment, or that he believed
his clamp-suture was inapplicable under such circumstances.
It is only through his followers that attention was first directed to this most important matter.

Again, Dr. Sims was almost wholly mistaken in the estimate he placed on the value of his self-retaining catheter.
Subsequent experience with it in the hands of other surgeons
proved that it was troublesome to manage, caused cystitis,
endangered the success of the method as a whole, proved inapplicable in a large proportion of cases, and, taken all in all,
was far inferior to the male (English) elastic catheter, when
any catheter at all was required.

Therefore, from all that has been said up to this point in
the discussion of the subject, it may be fairly stated that Dr.
Sims's attention was almost exclusively directed to the treatment, with his clamp-suture, of that simple class of fistules
alone known as vesico-vaginal, when the lesion was situated
at or near the center of the vesico-vaginal septum, as his Fig.

2 illustrates on a preceding page. Here the adjustment of
the apparatus was easy, and the clamps could always burrow
smoothly and uniformly into the tissues, as insisted upon by
him, provided there were no cicatricial contractions or inodular masses occupying the borders of the fistule. In transversely oval fistules thus favorably situated, with diameters
not exceeding an inch or an inch and a quarter, it was possible to secure with it and his self-retaining catheter a fair
degree of success. The proof of this limited adaptation of
the clamp-suture is found not only in Dr. Sims's own individual practice, but in that of nearly all of his followers, including (in the chronological order of cases treated by them)
the names of Sims and Bozeman, then of Montgomery, Ala.,
jointly, and Bozeman individually; Baker Brown, Mussey,
Thomas, Pope, Buck, Williams, Mettauer, Ash, Kollock,
Wragg, and Finnell.

It is important to state here that all the cases reported,
treated and not treated, by the above-named surgeons, be-
longed to the three classes of vesico-vaginal, urethro-vesico-
vaginal, and vesico-utero-vaginal fistules, with the exception
of a recto-vaginal fistule which was operated upon and cured
by Dr. R. D. Mussey, of Cincinnati, Ohio.

In order now to point out particularly the peculiarities
and relations of these three important lesions, and show the
precise mechanism of the clamp-suture, with the limitations
of its successful application in the several classes named, it
will be necessary to refer to the two original illustrations,
Figs. 4 and 5.

The two figures both represent fistules at the center of
the vesico-vaginal septum, the most common form and situation of the class of vesico-vaginal fistules, which are both
shown to be closed by a transverse application of the clamp-
suture similar to that illustrated by Dr. Sims (Fig. 2), but on
a reduced scale. Below the seat of these two fistules thus
closed with the clamp-suture are seen, at the junction of the
trigone of the bladder with the urethra, two fistules unclosed,
which belong to the class of urethro-vesico-vaginal fistules—

one a longitudinal slit (Fig. 4), unattended with loss of tissue
in either structure implicated, and the other (Fig. 5) a transversely oval opening, attended with loss of tissue in both
structures. These are the simplest forms of this class of

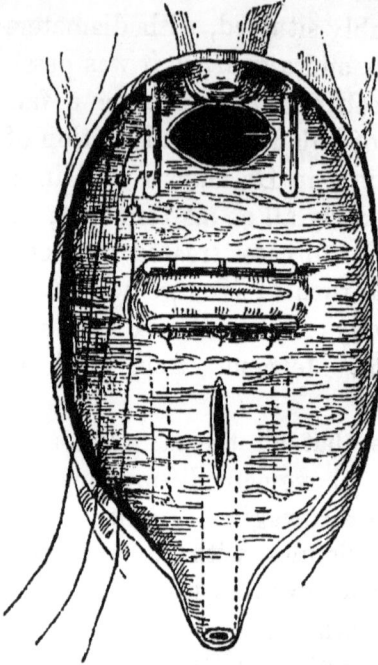 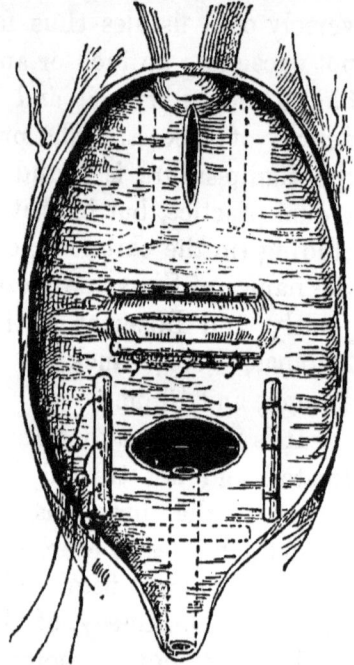

Fig. 4.   Fig. 5.

fistules.   In the first, the relative positions of the clamps, in
longitudinal outline, show the possibility of easily closing
the fistule ; but, in the second, the actual longitudinal positions of the clamps, with wires and perforated shot in readiness, show the impossibility of it, because the form of the
lesion, and the slight elasticity of the structures below within
the pubic arch, oppose the required mechanism of the clamps.
Here, then, parallel approximation could not be effected, or
their uniform burrowing into the tissues take place, without
serious damage to the structures on account of the underlying pubic bones.   For the application to the latter form of
fistules, therefore, the only other alternative would be to
change the positions of the two clamps to the sides of the

fistule and place them in a transverse relationship, as shown by the lower clamp on the closed vesico-vaginal fistule, and the clamp in dotted outline standing across the urethra. By such a mechanism of the clamps, coaptation of the borders of the fistule would be possible; not, however, by equal approximation of both borders, for the reasons before stated, but by stretching the tissues of the superior border of the fistule, in which alone any elasticity resides. As to the other requisite of the mechanism of the clamps always insisted upon by Dr. Sims—the burrowing into the underlying tissues —it is easy to see what the effect of the lower one would be upon the urethra compressed against the pubic arch. It would simply be cut in two and a urethro-vaginal fistule would be the result. With this explanation of the mechanism of the clamp-suture in a possible and impossible application of it, in the forms of the class of urethro-vesico-vaginal fistule illustrated, there will be no difficulty in imagining the increase of the defectiveness and dangers of the method, from the gradual augmentation of the size of the fistule, whether in one or more directions. Such a loss of tissue, it must not be forgotten, is liable to extend both longitudinally and transversely, sometimes involving the greater part or the whole of the urethra, on the one hand, and, on the other, the vesico-vaginal septum, together with a part or the whole of the infra-vaginal portion of the cervix uteri.

Let us next direct our attention beyond the seat of the two fistules, closed to the junction of the *bas-fond* of the bladder with the cervix uteri. Here are seen, also, two unclosed fistules which belong to the class of vesico-utero-vaginal fistules. One (Fig. 5) a longitudinal slit, unattended with loss of tissue in either structure implicated, and the other (Fig. 4) a transversely oval opening, attended with loss of tissue only in the *bas-fond* of the bladder. These are likewise the simplest forms of this class of fistules. In the first, the relative positions of the clamps in longitudinal outline, with their upper ends resting against the sides of the anterior lip of the cervix uteri, show the possibility of

easily closing the fistule, but, in the second, the actual longitudinal positions of the clamps and sutures show the impossibility of it, because the form of the lesion, the slight
transverse elasticity of the structures, and the position of the
somewhat solid anterior lip of the cervix uteri between the
upper ends of the clamps, all oppose the one essential ele-
ment of the mechanism—to wit, their parallel approximation.
The uniform burrowing of the clamps—the other requisite—
however, is possible here, but not without serious danger to
other important anatomical structures, notably the ureters.
In this form of the lesion, therefore, the only other alternative would be to introduce the same three sutures antero-
posteriorly, making the middle one traverse the anterior lip
of the cervix uteri in the median line, and the other two in
the borders of the fistule proper on either side of the cervix.
This being done, and the upper clamp placed on the upper
ends of the wires, across the cervix uteri, and the lower one
on the lower ends of the wires, in relation with the upper
clamp on the closed fistule, the next thing called for would
be the required adjustment of the apparatus, as illustrated
by its application to the vesico-vaginal fistule below.   What
would be the mechanism of the apparatus, from such an application of it, in such a relationship of the parts?   The
obvious and injurious result would be the undue pressure
of the clamp placed across the cervix uteri, supported only
at its middle, and mounted on a plane far above that of its
fellow of the opposite side.   The natural consequences of
such an unphilosophical application of the apparatus would
be to cause ulceration and the cutting across of the cervix
uteri, followed by hemorrhage and possibly cellulitis and
septic peritonitis, with permanent injury to the cervical canal,
should the patient be so fortunate as to escape with her life.
Still another grave consequence would be the almost certain
burrowing of the lower clamp into the vesico-vaginal septum,
and the opening of the bladder in its tract, simply, or by the
strangulation and sloughing of the included structures arising
from stress of the ascending uterus, thus cutting short the

prospect of permanent closure of the original fistule even by repetition of the procedure, should the patient be so fortunate as to escape with her life the disasters incident to a first trial.

Next imagine the augmentation of the size of the fistule by a more extended implication of a part or the whole of the infra-vaginal portion of the cervix uteri, and a part or the whole of the vesico-vaginal septum down to the urethra, even to the extent of destroying a part of the canal, all different phases or grades of implications that are constantly met with in practice, as I have often personally seen, and think of extending the application of this form of suture by lengthening the clamps to suit the diversified grades of lesion indicated. For the human mind to conceive a greater absurdity would seem clearly impossible.

How practical surgeons, in their experience with the clamp-suture, gradually approached the border-line of its efficiency and inefficiency, tried all sorts of expedients to accomplish cures which were impossible on account of the violation of natural laws involved in them, and invented all sorts of apologies for their disastrous failures, are interesting points of study. I propose, in my examination and analysis of the facts relating to the treatment of the several classes of lesions to which attention has been called, to present the views of each surgeon referred to, in his own words, so far as may be found practicable.

This brings us now to an examination, according to classification, of the peculiarities of fistules treated with the clamp-suture in the United States and England, during the period of sixteen years extending from 1845 to December, 1861, when the last operation with it, of which there is any account, was performed, by Dr. T. C. Finnell, of New York.

. In this period are comprised all the fistules and injuries incident to parturition, and the results of their treatment with the clamp-suture, reported by Dr. Sims and the different surgeons before enumerated. The number of cases constituting the first series was thirty-eight, and they presented forty-three fistules and injuries belonging to six classes—twenty-four vesico-vaginal fistules, seven urethro-vesico-vaginal fistules, six vesico-utero-vaginal fistules, two urethro-vaginal fistules, two recto-vaginal fistules, and two lacerations of the perineum.

The cases admitted into the Woman's Hospital of the State of New York, and treated individually by Dr. Sims with the clamp-suture, from May, 1855, to May, 1856, when he abandoned this form of suture, are comprised, as before stated, in the second series. The number also amounted to thirty-seven, in which there were forty-two fistules and injuries belonging to five classes—seventeen vesico-vaginal fistules, seven urethro-vesico-vaginal fistules, eight vesico-utero-vaginal fistules, five recto-vaginal fistules, and five lacerations of the perineum. The number of cases in this second series, and the classification of the same in one year, are thus shown to be, by an extraordinary coincidence, almost precisely the same as those given in the first series, the treatment of which extended through a period of sixteen years, and, what is no less remarkable, the results of treatment in this second series vary but little from those of the first, as will hereafter be shown.

There is no evidence to be found, in connection with this second series of cases in the Woman's Hospital, that Dr. T. A. Emmet, the successor in 1862 of Dr. Sims, ever performed an operation with the clamp-suture, but his labors during the period named, beginning with the opening of the hospital, May 1, 1855, and showing his faithful record of the histories and peculiarities of the cases of this series, are not without great practical value in a statistical point of view. For this record, Dr. Emmet is certainly entitled to the highest credit from the profession, and I for my part heartily acknowledge this deep sense of obligation to him, since without it the individual efforts of Dr. Sims in this institution at that period, supported as they were by the resources of the great State of New York, and encouraged by the sympathies and sacrifices of a few noble women, would have been entirely lost to science, whatever may now be thought of their philosophy or usefulness.

Class of Vesico-vaginal Fistules.

CASES I–III.—*First Three Vesico-vaginal Fistules cured with the Clamp-Suture—Lesions situated at or near the Center of the Vesico-vaginal Septum—No Complications present— Forty Operations performed, mostly experimental, before the Method was perfected and the Cures completed.*

Anacha, Lucy, and Betsy, all colored, were the first three women treated by Dr. Sims, in Montgomery, Ala., from 1845 to June, 1849, with his various modifications of the old quill-suture, and, finally, with his perfected clamp-suture. They were all completely cured eventually ; the three having undergone from first to last no less than forty operations in all. From the best information that can be gathered from the various published sources extant, regarding the peculiarities of these cases, the writer is led to conclude that the fistules in the outset were all of small size and favorably situated, at or about the center of the vesico-vaginal septum, in vaginas otherwise normal. These three cases are of peculiar historical interest, from the great number of operations they underwent, and the gratifying results that were finally realized. It is to be regretted that Dr. Sims never made a detailed report of them.

CASE IV.—*Vesico-vaginal Fistule—Lesion Small, situated near the Center of the Vesico-vaginal Septum—No Complications present—One Operation with the Clamp-Suture—Self-retaining Catheter caused Inflammation of Urethra, and had to be removed on the Fourth Day—Clamps removed on Ninth Day, and found burrowed into the Tissues, almost out of Sight —First Operation Successful.*

Ann McKee,[1] colored, aged sixteen, came under Dr. Sims's care in the autumn of 1849, and presented a transversely oval fistule situated just below the center of the vesico-vaginal septum, as shown by Fig. 6, copied from his original illustration. Dr. Sims operated upon the case October 25, 1849, with his

---

[1] See Case I, *New York Med. Gazette*, vol. v, January, 1854.

clamp-suture, using three points of silver wire, and, in the after-treatment, his self-retaining catheter.

He states that on the fourth day *the urethra became much inflamed and swollen, when the catheter had to be removed entirely* and the patient allowed to pass the urine naturally. An examination on the seventh day *showed the clamps to be completely hidden in the tissues from burrowing, only the projecting ends of the wires and perforated shot being visible* (italics by the writer). The apparatus was removed on the ninth day. Of the condition of the cicatrix on the eleventh day Dr. Sims says : "The sulci on each side of it made by the clamps were filled up by granulations, while the cicatrix, which two days ago was so compact as scarcely to be visible, is now considerably *widened, thinned, and depressed below the vaginal surface,* and evidently seems to be on the point of giving way" (italics his). He afterward remarks : "This was the first case I had cured by a single operation, and I felt great satisfaction at the result, particularly as it was obtained under such unfavorable circumstances."

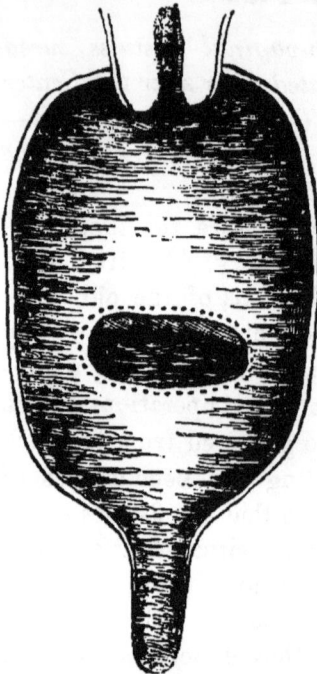
Fig. 6.

CASE V. — *Vesico-vaginal Fistule—Situation same as in Preceding Case, but Size Larger—No Complications present— Patient very large, and could not bear the Knee-Elbow Position—Operation with Clamp-Suture performed on the Left Side—Clamps removed on the Sixth Day, and found burrowed out of Sight in the Substance of the Bladder—Cicatrization of the Sulci thus produced nearly caused Reproduction of the Fistule—First Operation successful.*

Mrs. A. F.,[1] aged forty, quite stout, and weighing nearly two hundred pounds, applied to Dr. Sims for treatment. He

[1] See Case II, *op. cit.*

says : "Fistula was considerably larger than the one first described, but occupied precisely the same relative position with regard to other parts." He operated with the clamp-suture on November 12, 1849, when three points of suture were used. Owing to the inability of the patient to bear the *knee-elbow position,* Dr. Sims placed her on the *left side* for the operation, of which he thus speaks :

"Placed on her left side, with the thighs well flexed on the abdomen, the nates forcibly pulled upward and backward, the lever-speculum was introduced and the parts brought into view, which was accomplished more easily than I anticipated, but did not show the fistula so well as when the proper position on the knees is resorted to. However, I managed to get through with the different stages of the operation with tolerable ease. . . .

"On the sixth day the clamps were removed. They were *buried in the substance of the bladder, and entirely hidden from view, the leaden knots alone being visible.* The fistula seemed to be accurately and perfectly closed ; the line of union being scarcely perceptible [italicized by the writer]. . . .

"It [the cicatrix] underwent precisely the same changes as noticed in the former case, only to a greater degree : viz., *a stretching, thinning, and depression,* which gradually disappeared, the cicatrix then becoming smooth and regular [italicized by him].

"It follows, then, that three or four days is not long enough for the suture apparatus to remain, because the fistula has always been reproduced after its removal ; and that seven or eight days is not sufficient, because there is great danger of the same accident. My large experience has demonstrated the fact that about twelve days is the proper length of time for the clamp-suture to remain in the tissues. It is evidently unsafe to remove it sooner, and it may remain till the fifteenth day with impunity, but a longer time is altogether unnecessary."

CASE VI.—*Vesico-vaginal Fistule—Situation near Center of Vesico-vaginal Septum—Size very Small, and Direction through the Tissues Valvular—No Complications present— First Operation with Clamp-Suture successful.*

Mrs. H.[1] applied to Dr. Sims for the treatment of a small
fistule situated in the upper part of the trigone of the bladder,
as seen in the accompanying illustration, Fig. 7, and thus described by him : "The fistulous opening was just above the
neck of the bladder, a little to the right of the mesial line, and
altogether favorable for a successful operation.   It ran diag-

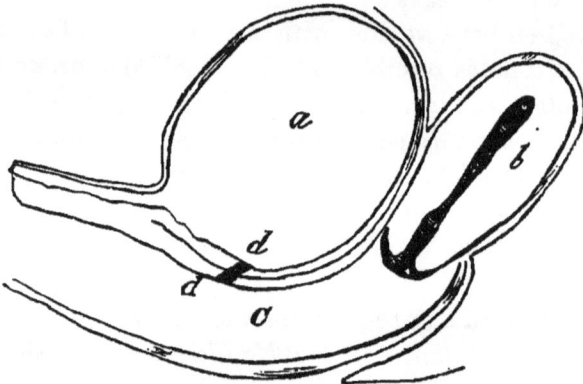

Fig. 7.

onally through the walls of the bladder, thus forming a sort
of sinuous canal of a valvular character."   Dr. Sims operated
upon the case February 2, 1853, using two points of suture
with his clamps, and completed the cure at a single operation.
Suture apparatus removed on the thirteenth day.   (Illustration
copied.)

CASE VII.— *Vesico-vaginal Fistule without Loss of Tissue,
being the Result of Vesico-vaginal Lithotomy—Direction of
Incision longitudinal—Situation in Trigone of Bladder—Cal-
culus, Size of a Partridge's Egg—Easily seized and removed—
Vagina naturally Small, but otherwise Normal—Eight or ten
Operations with the Clamp-Suture— Conversion of the Original
Incision into a Round Opening, the Size of the Index-Finger,
and the Establishment of a Urethro-vesico-vaginal Fistule with
Complete Obliteration at the Same Point of the Urethral Canal,
and Extensive Cicatricial Surfaces around both Fistules, all
Results of the repeated cutting away of the Tissues and slough-
ing out of the Suture Apparatus—Patient discharged incurable.*

[1] *New York Medical Times*, May, 1854, and *American Journal of the Medical Sciences*, vol. xxviii, p. 283, July, 1854.

Lavinia Boudurant, colored, aged thirteen, applied to Dr. Sims for treatment, on account of a calculus in the bladder, in the spring of 1850. The incision made for the removal of the stone was in the median line, and extended upward from a point near the junction of the urethra with the trigone of the bladder. It was about three quarters of an inch in length, and consequently extended slightly into the *bas-fond* of the bladder. The calculus was seized with forceps and removed through this opening. As soon as the bladder was cleansed of blood, Dr. Sims made a longitudinal application of his clamp-suture, the position of the clamps being the same as shown by dotted lines in the diagram, Fig. 4, illustrating a urethro-vesico-vaginal fistule unattended with loss of tissue. The result of this application of the clamps proved a total failure. I was present and assisted in the operation. During the next eighteen months or two years, the patient underwent, without success, eight or ten similar operations, in many of which I also assisted. The final result was the conversion of the original straight incision in the trigone of the bladder into a transversely oval vesico-vaginal fistule,

from the repeated paring away of the tissues, and the ulcerating out of the suture apparatus. There was established also an additional complication from the same causes, a urethro-vesico-vaginal fistule about half an inch from the lower border of the existing vesico-vaginal one, and a complete obliteration of the urethral canal at the seat of the accidental opening. Over the obliterated portion of the urethra, and around the borders of each fistule, were to be seen extensive surfaces of a

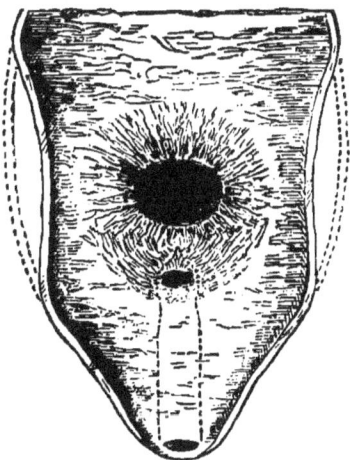

Fig. 8.

cicatricial or inodular tissue, resulting also from the repeated cutting out of the clamps, as shown by the wavy lines in the accompanying illustration (Fig. 8). The relation of the two fistules, as well as the obliterated point of the urethra between them, are also shown.

No report of this case was ever made by Dr. Sims.

Some six or seven years after this patient was discharged by Dr. Sims, she applied to me for further treatment (January 18, 1858), when both of her fistules, together with the stricture of the urethra, as above described, were completely cured at two operations by gradual preparatory treatment, and the *button-suture*, as will be more fully described hereafter, in the consideration of the class of urethro-vesico-vaginal fistules.

CASE VIII.— *Vesico-vaginal Fistule—Situation of the Lesion below the Center of the Vesico-vaginal Septum—Transversely Oval and of Medium Size—No Complications present —Ten or more Operations with the Clamp-Suture—Closure of the Fistule in the Middle, leaving two Angular Openings—Patient abandoned for a Time uncured.*

Delia, colored, aged twenty-three, Dr. Sims's own servant. She began to receive treatment from Dr. Sims in the spring of 1850, and this was continued from that time up to March, 1853. Now becoming associated with Dr. Sims as partner, I had the opportunity of seeing the exact stage of advancement in the treatment of the case. Having also been present and assisted in some of the many operations previously performed by Dr. Sims, I had become thoroughly acquainted with the difficulties pertaining to the case. The fistule originally occupied a low and very accessible position in the vesico-vaginal septum, and extended transversely, but further to the right of the median line than to the left. It was in the outset oval in outline, and measured perhaps an inch and a quarter in its longest diameter. During the period the patient was under Dr. Sims's treatment, she underwent ten or more operations, according to her own account. Dr. Sims stated to me, regarding the previous history of his treatment, that by his first two or three operations he succeeded in closing the fistule in the middle and narrowing it down to two small angular openings, which had since defied all efforts to complete the cure.

On or about May 20, 1853, Dr. Sims performed his last operation, which was a double one, and consisted in applying a pair of clamps to each remaining fistule. He left the after-treatment to me, this being only a few days before his own departure from Montgomery for New York. The result of the operation was a total failure, both pairs of clamps cutting out. No report of the case was ever made by Dr. Sims. The woman remained in this condition until the autumn of 1855, when she applied to me for further treatment. Both fistùles were completely closed, each at a single operation, by means of the button-suture. The case will be referred to again and illustrated in another connection.

CASE IX.— *Vesico-vaginal Fistule—Size Small, and Situation near the Cervix Uteri, and to the left of the Median Line— Cicatricial Contraction of the Left Wall of the Vagina with Distortion of the Organ opposite the same Point—Complications not treated—Three Operations with the Clamp-Suture for Closure of Fistule—All failed from the early cutting out of the Left Clamp—Dr. Sims's Lever-Speculum found to be too short to expose the Fistule—Important Modification of this Instrument—Patient first discharged uncured, and finally considered incurable, by the Clamp-Suture.*

Julia McDuffie, colored, aged twenty. She first came under observation early in March, 1853, and was treated jointly by Dr. Sims and myself, this being the first new case in our practice after we became associated as partners. The fistule was about the size of a No. 6 catheter, and was situated near the cervix uteri, about midway between the median line and left lateral wall of the vagina. Between it and the wall of the vagina, the parts showed the effects of direct injury, which had resulted in slight contraction of the canal at this point, together with a thickening and elevation of the corresponding border of the fistule to a plane above that of its fellow of the opposite side.

Owing to the distortion of the vagina at this point, and the shortness of the lever-speculum as improved by Dr. Sims, great difficulty attended the effort of displaying the fistule in the knee-elbow position. The anterior wall of the vagina, being thus drawn toward the posterior, and restrained in its movements, could not drop to the usual position when the speculum was introduced and air admitted into the organ, as always insisted upon by Dr. Sims as an important principle. Gravitation of the pelvic and abdominal viscera took place as usual, but the anterior wall of the vagina remained in its more or less restrained relationship with the posterior, thus preventing exposure of the fistule, as before stated. Nevertheless, on or about March 15, 1853, Dr. Sims performed his operation with the clamp-suture. I held the speculum, and of course saw the complication present, and realized fully the disadvantages of the short blade of the speculum for displaying the fistule. The nearness of the opening to the anterior lip of the cervix uteri precluded the possibility of making a transverse adjustment of the apparatus, even had the parts been in a normal state. Under such circumstances a longitudinal application became the only alternative, and this necessitated the placing of the left clamp upon the hardened and unyielding border of the fistule described, and of the right, upon the soft and elastic one.

Two points of suture were used. Fig. 9 illustrates the closure of the fistule and the apparatus in position, together with the cicatricial contraction and distortion of the vagina on the left side.

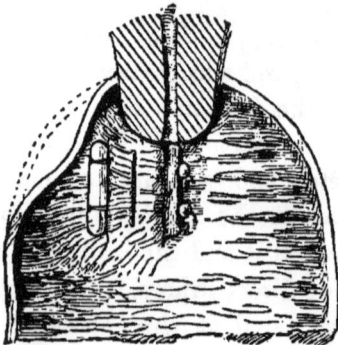
Fig. 9.

The left clamp, as shown, rested on a plane higher than its fellow of the opposite side, and, instead of sinking into the tissues to reach an easy, even point of adjustment, it caused ulceration, and cut its way down, in the course of the after-treatment, to the required level, with consequent strangulation and sloughing of the included structures; thus resulting in an increase in the size of the original opening.

Under the same difficulties with regard to exposure of the fistule, I performed the same operation June 1, 1853, and with precisely the same unfortunate result.

In both of these operations, the patient showed great suffering, and in her struggles became quite exhausted at times. Finally, not being able to maintain the knee-elbow position, she sank into that of the knee-face, in which the procedure was completed, as usual under such circumstances.

The general health of the patient suffered very much from these operations, and she was consequently sent home with no encouragement whatever to expect an ultimate cure.

No report by Dr. Sims of this case, or his operation, was ever made. Nearly two years afterward, however, the patient returned to me for further treatment. I will speak of the subsequent operations and final result in another connection.

Having observed the defectiveness of Dr. Sims's form of the lever-speculum, as employed in these two operations, it occurred to me that the instrument might be greatly improved for the treatment of all cases having the complication above described. In June, 1853, I submitted my plan of modification of the instrument to a jeweler,[1] upon whom I was dependent at that time for all such impromptu work. The result was the embodiment of all my proposed alterations, which proved most satisfactory. The accompanying cuts show the original forms of the two instruments—Fig. 10 Sims's, and Fig. 11 Bozeman's.

The objects of these alterations in the form of Dr. Sims's speculum, without regard to aid from atmospheric pressure, and believed to be called for in this case, were threefold :

1. To increase the length of the blade of the instrument from two inches and a half, as described by Dr. Sims, to about four inches, so as to make it extend the whole length of the posterior wall of the vagina, thus making it pass into or beyond the point of cicatricial contraction.

2. To make the heel of the blade narrower, and the distal extremity wider, so as to insure greater elevation of the perineum, and consequently more forcible expansion of the cicatricially contracted portion of the vagina, necessary for exposure of the co-existing fistule.

3. To place the handle of the instrument at such an angle to the blade, 75°, that it could be easily held in the right hand of the assistant, with the forearm resting over the sacrum of the patient, thus giving the required adaptation of

---

[1] John Bates, of Montgomery, Ala.

the blade to the entire rectal wall of the vagina without fatigue of the arm, as from the elevated and awkward angle of the elbow requisite in the use of Dr. Sims's form of the instrument. To show that all of these alterations were philo-

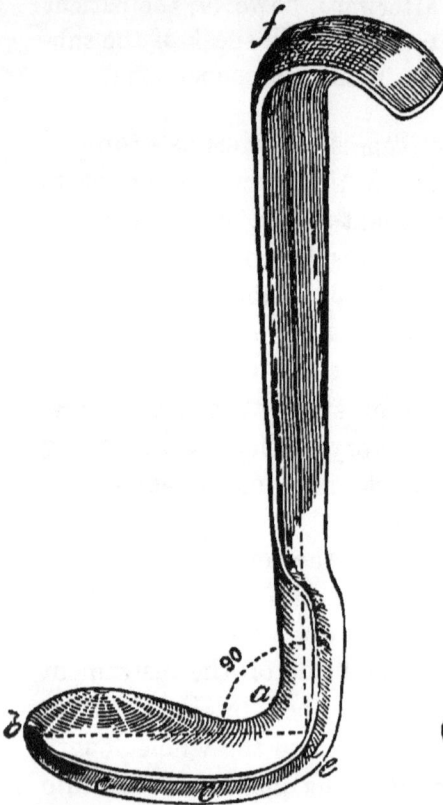

Fig. 10.

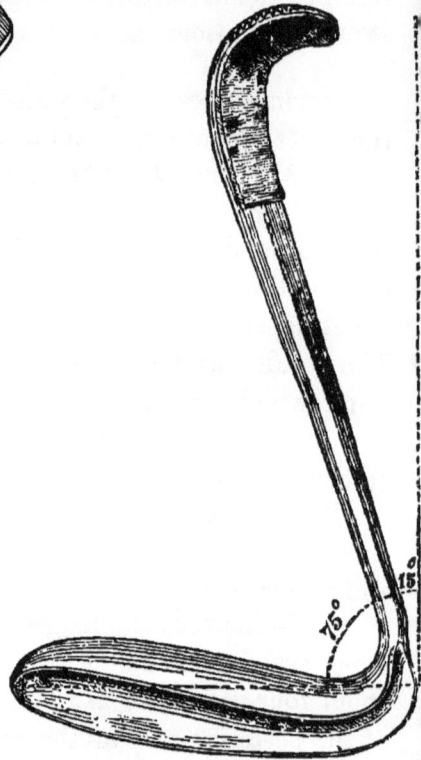

Fig. 11.

sophical, and the objects of them fully attained, I will only state the fact that my pattern of the instrument, as above shown, superseded in my hands entirely that of Dr. Sims, which was intended originally for the simple purpose of elevating the perineum and securing the admission of air, thought by him to be sufficient for the distension of the vagina.

CASE X.— *Vesico-vaginal Fistule—Situation supposed to have been favorable in the Vesico-vaginal Septum—Important Modification of the Clamp-Suture—First Operation with it successful.*

Dr. Mussey, in his report[1] of the first successful operation for recto-vaginal fistule, by an important modification of the clamp-suture, April 20, 1853, incidentally refers to an unreported case · of vesico-vaginal fistule operated upon by a surgeon in Ohio, who had also modified the clamp-suture in a somewhat similar manner to that proposed by himself. · He says : "Dr. Thomas, in the eastern part of Ohio, now of Pittsburgh, Pa., who treated a case of vesico-vaginal fistula with entire success, placed his stitches in the clamp-suture about the fifth of an inch apart. The wire which I employed in the recto-vaginal fistula was not far from twice the diameter of a horse-hair." This case of recto-vaginal fistule will be introduced in its appropriate place in the consideration of this class. Although the situation, size, and form of the fistule in Dr. Thomas's case were not stated by Dr. Mussey, the inference may be fairly made, from the success of the operation, that the lesion occupied the usual position at or near the center of the vesico-vaginal septum.

CASES XI–XIII.—*Three Vesico-vaginal Fistules—First one of Medium Size, and situated near the Center of the Vesico-vaginal Septum—No Complications present on the Anterior Wall of the Vagina, but upon the Posterior existed a few Cicatricial Bands— Complication not treated—First Operation with Clamp-Suture successful—Self-retaining Catheter caused Cystitis, and its Use had to be discontinued—Fistules in Second and Third Cases large, but supposed to have been favorably situated in the Vesico-vaginal Septum — Grave Cicatricial Contractions of the Vagina present—Complications not treated— Operated upon by Heated Wire and Ordinary Suture, and by the Methods of Hayward, Jobert, and Sims, but all failed—Both Cases discharged as incurable.*

Mary Porch, aged thirty, came under the care of Dr. Charles A. Pope,[2] of St. Louis, in the autumn of 1853, presenting a fistule at the center of the vesico-vaginal septum, with a transverse diameter of an inch and a quarter. There were slight cicatricial contractions upon the posterior vaginal wall, and calcareous incrustations and excoriations of the external parts were

---

[1] *American Journal of the Medical Sciences*, vol. xxvii, Oct., 1853.
[2] *St. Louis Med. and Surg. Jour.*, vol. xii, p. 401, Aug., 1854.

also present.   On December 3d, Dr. Pope proceeded to operate
with the clamp-suture, and was entirely successful at the first
trial.   He states that the *self-retaining catheter of Dr.
Sims, in the after-treatment, caused cystitis, and its use had to be discontinued.*   He concludes his report of the case with an allu-
sion to two other cases, treated by the same method, but prov-
ing unsuccessful on account of the complication of cicatricial
contractions of the vagina.   As showing the gravity of such
complications, and how they were regarded by Dr. Sims at
this stage of his experience with the clamp-suture, the writer
will quote Dr. Pope's own words.   He says :

"I have tried various modes of relief in these distressing
cases of vesico-vaginal fistulæ, as the heated wire, the ordinary
suture with freshened edges, Hayward's as well as Jobert's
methods, and in three instances Sims's operation.   Partial benefit occurred in almost every case.   The two former instances, in
which I failed by Sims's operation, *were not favorable cases,
owing to their great size and the accompanying coarctations of
the vagina.   In describing one of these cases to Dr Sims himself, whom I had the pleasure of meeting at the American Medical Association, held in Richmond, Va. (1854), he stated that he
would not have undertaken an operation for its relief.*   [Italics
by the writer.]   Cures of vesico-vaginal fistula have doubtlessly
been effected by other means, but the success in my last case
was so easily and completely attained that I must confess my
decided preference for the operation adopted.   Too much
praise can not be awarded Dr. Sims for his persevering and in-
genious efforts in this department."

CASE XIV.— *Vesico-vaginal Fistule—Situation near the
Center of the Septum, and Size Small—No Complications
present—Lithotomy Position, and Anesthesia used in the
Operation—Jacobson's Lithotrite applied to expose the Fist-
ule—Operation for Closure of the Same by an important
Modification of the Clamp-Suture—Employment of Silver
Wire and Flat Clamps instead of Round Ones, and of Two
Interrupted Silver Wires, each secured independently with
Perforated Shot—First Use of Interrupted Silver - Wire Su-
tures secured in this Way—Anterior Clamp burrowed into the
Tissues, leaving an ulcerated Groove—Fistule completely closed.*

Mary Harty, aged twenty-eight, came under the care of Dr. Gurdon Buck,[1] in the New York Hospital, July 4, 1854. The fistule was situated just below the center of the vesico-vaginal septum, and was of the size of the index-finger. Dr. Buck operated on this case on July 13, 1854, placing the patient in the lithotomy *position, and using an anesthetic.* Of the procedure adopted, which was an important modification of Dr. Sims's method, he says :

" A Jacobson's lithotrite answered a most useful purpose in bringing within reach the fistulous opening, and keeping the surrounding vesico-vaginal wall on the stretch, thus very much facilitating the subsequent steps of the operation. This instrument resembles in form an ordinary catheter with a short curve. The curve, when the instrument is opened, is converted into a pointed hook, or noose. It was introduced closed per urethram into the bladder and then opened. By elevating the handle of the instrument toward the abdomen, the loop was depressed against the base of the bladder, forcing it downward into the vagina, and forward toward the vulva. The fistule being thus brought within reach, its edges are pared away, so as to render the longest diameter of the opening transverse."

The fistule having been thus exposed, and its edges pared, Dr. Buck introduced six silver sutures, and then secured them with "a narrow, flat strip of lead, called a clamp," and perforated shot. *Only the four middle wires were secured with the clamps and shot. The two end ones were fastened independently by simply running down on each one of them a perforated shot, and compressing it.* The clamps and sutures were removed on the fourteenth day, and closure of the fistule found complete. The *anterior clamp had burrowed into the tissues some, leaving in its site an ulcerated groove.* (Italics by the writer.)

The particulars in which Dr. Buck departed from Dr. Sims's procedure may be summed up as follows :

1. The patient was placed in the lithotomy position, instead of the knee-elbow.

2. An anesthetic was used.

3. Jacobson's lithotrite was used for displaying the fistule, instead of the lever-speculum.

[1] *New York Journal of Medicine,* vol. iv, October, 1854.

4. A greater number of sutures were used, and the two end ones were secured independently of the clamps, as interrupted sutures, by compressing on them perforated shot.

5. Narrow, flat clamps were used, instead of small, round ones, preferred by Dr. Sims to facilitate their burrowing into the tissues.

CASE XV.— *Vesico-vaginal Fistule—Situation at or near the Center of the Septum, and of a Size to admit Two Fingers with Longest Diameter transverse—No Complications present— Two Operations with the Clamp-Suture—In Second Operation the Apparatus found burrowed into the Tissues—Closure of Fistule successful.*

Mrs. R. came under the care of Dr. A. V. Williams,[1] of New York, in the autumn of 1854, presenting a fistule near the center of the vesico-vaginal septum, in a vagina otherwise normal. It was large enough to admit two fingers. Dr. Williams performed the operation, "as recommended by Dr. Sims," October 14, 1854. Everything progressed well until the fifth day, when the escape of urine per vaginam was discovered. Now, "on examination it was found *ulceration had taken place at one end of the clamps*, probably from their having been applied too firmly. It may here be remarked that *the proper application of the clamps is one of the nicest points of the operation: if applied too loosely, urine will escape; if too tight, they will ulcerate. It is difficult to state the degree of pressure necessary; it is a matter for the exercise of judgment on the part of the operator.* It perhaps may do to suggest that, if the clean edges of the cut surfaces are brought into exact coaptation it will answer, as the swelling, of the parts will then keep them well together. The condition of the clamps was always exactly as stated by Dr. Sims, and need not here be repeated."

The clamps were removed on the eleventh day, when the fistule was found to be reduced to the size of one finger, the operation having practically failed.

Dr. Williams performed a second operation, using the same form of suture, in December, 1854. He removed the apparatus this time on the fourteenth day, finding it "*lying seemingly enclosed in a new mucous surface"* ; but the result was a complete closure of the fistule. (Italics by the writer.)

CASE XVI.— *Vesico-vaginal Fistule—Situation at or near the Center of the Septum, and Size half an inch in Diameter —No Complications present—One Operation with the Clamp-Suture—In the After-treatment, the Perforations in the Self-retaining Catheter became closed by Projections into them of the Mucous Coat of the Bladder—Closure of the Fistule successful.*

A colored woman, aged twenty-three, was placed under the care of Dr. W. C. Ashe,[1] of Demopolis, Ala., in the spring of 1855. No statement of the seat or form of the fistule is made, but it is said to have been half an inch in diameter. From the meager report of the details of the case, and the promptness with which it was cured with the clamp-suture at a single operation, it is safe to say that the fistule occupied a favorable position for the burrowing of the clamps, at or near the center of the vesico-vaginal septum. The after-treatment was conducted by Dr. Ruffin, who had trouble with the self-retaining catheter, as may be inferred from the following statement : "He found that granulations would shoot rapidly into the foramina of the catheter so as to render its removal indispensable to the free discharge of urine."

The operation was performed in March, 1855, and the patient discharged cured.

CASE XVII. — *Three Fistules, one Vesico-vaginal, one Urethro-vesico-vaginal, and one Urethro-vaginal—Situation of Vesico-vaginal Fistule near the Center of the Septum— Direction Longitudinal and of a Size to admit Point of Index-Finger—Cicatricial Contraction of the Vagina to the same estimated Size of the Fistule—Alkaline Urine and Extensive Excoriations of the Internal and External Genital Parts— First Successful Employment jointly of Bozeman's Improved Lever-Speculum, of his Supported Knee-Chest Position, and of his Gradual Preparatory Treatment—Very close Relationship of the Vesico-vaginal and the Urethro-vesico-vaginal Fistule—Only possible to close one Opening at a Time with the Clamp-Suture—Operated first upon the Former—Result, a*

*Complete Failure from the sloughing out of the Apparatus—
Causes of the Disaster, Hardness of the Tissues, and Poisonous
Effects of the Urine upon the Denuded Edges of the Fistule,
flowing into the Vagina through the Neighboring Fistule—
Case now considered incurable unless Protection against the
Evil Effects of the Urine could in some Way be Secured—In-
vention of the Button-Suture made for this Purpose, about a
Month afterward.*

Matilda Stamper,[1] colored, aged twenty-one, came under
my care in Montgomery, Ala., February 9, 1855. Description
at the time of admission as follows : " Found the vagina very
much contracted by indurated bands extending across it. One
just below the cervix uteri occasioned such narrowing of the
canal that the point of the index-finger could scarcely be passed
through it. On the posterior side of the organ the induration
and contraction were greatest, giving rise to considerable short-
ening of the canal, and drawing in the labium pudendi of the
right side. Communicating with the urethra, very near the
meatus, there was a small opening ; further back, just across
the beginning or root of the urethra, was situated another,
about three quarters of an inch in length and, of course, communicating with the bladder. About half an inch above this
last, and to the extreme right, was situated still another opening about the same size. These two last, one having its longest diameter transverse, and the other longitudinal, represented
two sides of a square.

"In attempting now to pass a catheter through the urethra
into the bladder, I found great difficulty, owing to distortion
at its neck, caused by the anterior border of the fistule, situated
thus, being drawn up to the pubic bones.

(See Fig. 12, two thirds size [knee-chest position], introduced here to show the contraction and distortion of the vaginal tract, and the situations of the three classes of fistules
indicated. The dotted lines, seen running across the vesico-
vaginal septum at C, point to the upper and lower extremities
of the vesico-vaginal fistule situated to the right side, half an
inch from the median section. B stands in the breach of the

[1] See Case XVI, *New Orleans Med. and Surg. Jour.*, January, March, and
May, 1860.

urethro-vesico-vaginal fistule, formed at the expense of both
the trigone of the bladder and the root of the urethra, the end
of the latter being obliterated and drawn out of line with the
corresponding border of the fistule, and fixed behind the pubic
bones. A indicates the break between the vagina and urethra
just behind the meatus urinarius. B illustrates the point of

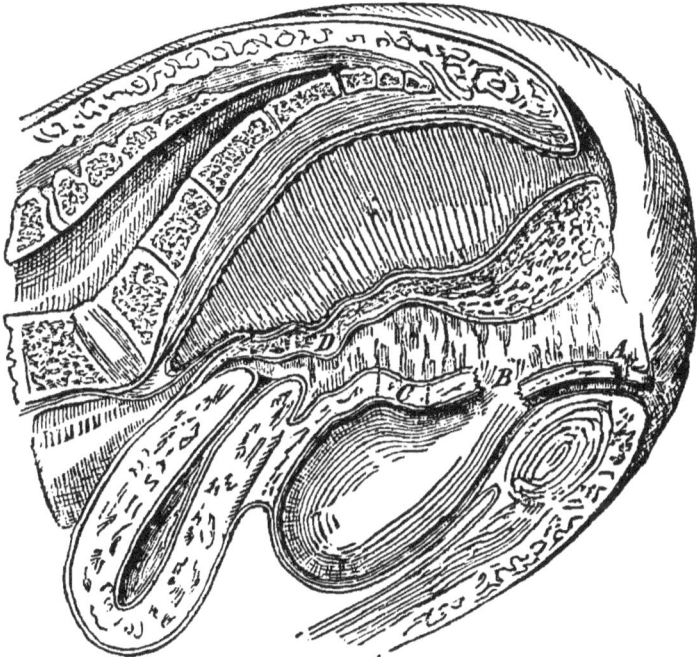

Fig. 12.

greatest contraction and distortion of the vaginal tract, it not
admitting there the point of the index-finger.)

"Having considered now the case in all its bearings, I
determined to make an application of Dr. Sims's 'clamp-suture,' this being the one I was at that time employing. Before
proceeding to the operation, however, the question arose in
my mind as to the possibility of closing both of the vesical
openings at once by two sets of clamps, this appearing to me
to be the preferable course. Upon a minute examination now
of the parts, with reference to the practicability of such a procedure, I was convinced that it could not be done, owing to the
narrowness of the intervening tissue, upon which both sets of

clamps would have to rest. Thus applied, one of each set of clamps would necessarily cross the other. Seeing this difficulty, therefore, I determined upon the only other alternative, which was to close one opening at a time. The upper one (the vesico-vaginal fistule) I selected for my first operation, thinking by this *to avoid, to some extent, the irritating effect of the urine passing through the lower opening. As a preparatory measure now for this operation, I had to make deep incisions in the contracting bands of the vagina, and then dilate the organ by the use of tents. This took up considerable time, and was the cause of much suffering to the patient, owing to the excessive irritability of the parts.*"

Fig. 13 illustrates the kind of tent or dilator which, after

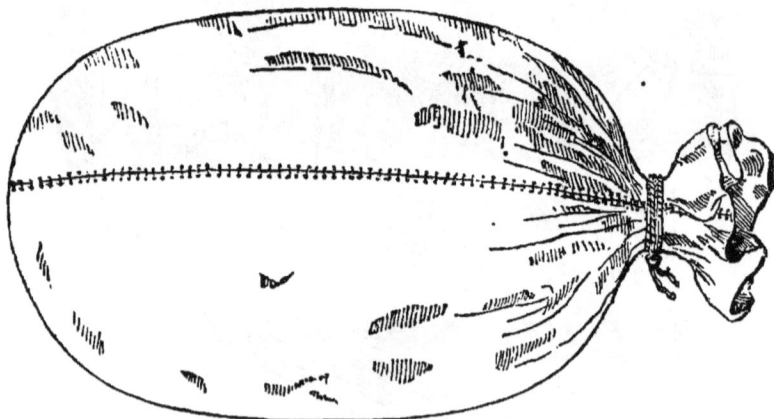

Fig. 13.

much experimentation and several failures, was finally adopted, with the necessary incisions, as the proper mode of *gradual preparatory treatment.*

It would be interesting here to point out the special advantages of this kind of sponge-dilator over that made of hard material (which could not be borne by this patient), but space does not permit. Suffice it to say, this bag of oil-silk, here represented two thirds size, is filled with torn pieces of coarse sponge, every piece being compressed separately, so as to give the whole the required firmness for easy introduction. This form of dilator is also far better and more manageable than the ordinary compressed sponge-tents shielded in the same.

manner, because, in the use of it, the exact amount of pressure needed can always be determined beforehand, a most important precaution. This is the size used in the case, the diameter being about an inch and three quarters (about forty-four millimetres). This was the limit of the dilatation reached in the case, after a little more than six weeks of persevering effort. But even with this limit of expansion of the vagina, there still remained a considerable degree of hardness and stiffness of the vaginal walls—a leathery condition, so to speak, with more or less persistent resiliency. My improved lever-speculum, used for displaying the cicatricial and contracted points in the vagina, was found to be very much restricted in its applicability. Owing to the implication of the rectal wall, the incisions here had to be made without the instrument. For making the required incisions, the employment of a properly adapted bivalve or dilating speculum for putting on the stretch cicatricially contracted bands would, no doubt, have contributed to a much higher degree of expansion of the vagina, and, consequently, a much more satisfactory display of all the fistules, than were attainable in the way described, but there was no such instrument in use at that time.

It is also important to mention here the fact that, during the stage of preparatory treatment, the patient bore badly the fatigue of the *knee-elbow* position, she having to change all the while from this to the very objectionable *knee-face* position, according to her fatigue or the severity of her sufferings. To obviate this unsteadiness of the patient, and insure greater safety and certainty in making the incisions, I resorted to the expedient, adopted in other cases for a year or so before, of placing her body in a horizontal position and supporting it there upon pillows, piled up one upon another, under the chest and head—the most comfortable and useful of all the anterior positions. By this plan, and a sufficient number of assistants to hold her upon the pillows, it was found quite possible to make her comfortable, and to secure the advantages of an anesthetic with safety. But, from the softness of the pillows, and their readiness to become disarranged attending the excitement of the anesthetic and the resistance of the patient, a bench of suitable height, surmounted by a firm cushion, was finally substituted for the former. This arrangement turned out to be a great improvement upon the pillows as a *chest and head support,* and afterward was always employed when an anesthetic was required. It finally became the sustaining part of what I described a few years later as my supporting and fixing apparatus for the *knee-chest position* without assistants. Attention will hereafter be directed specially to the superior advantages of this last improvement for overcoming the previously recognized necessity of kolpokleisis and for the performance of all operations upon the anterior wall of the vagina, and to a very large extent for those upon the posterior wall as well.

Fig. 14 shows the patient in this position, held by assistants

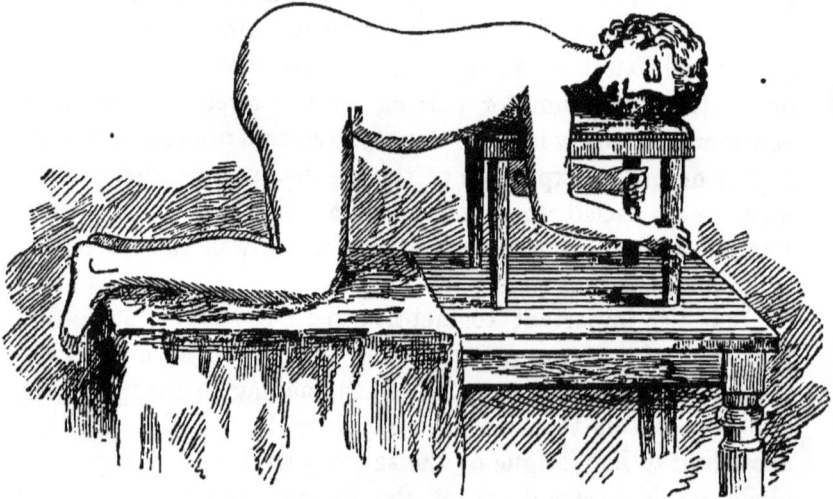

Fig. 14.

upon the cushioned bench, ready for the anesthetic and the operation for closure of the vesico-vaginal fistule, after completing the gradual preparatory treatment.

Present as assistants at this operation were Dr. W. C. Jackson, and two students of medicine, Mr. Hannon and Mr. Tarver, all of Montgomery, Ala.

Here follows a description of the operation and result :

" *Operation,* March 23, 1855.—Everything being as favorable as could be expected under the circumstances, the operation above indicated was performed. *Owing to the great induration and contraction of the parts, I encountered no little difficulty*

in going through with the different stages. Three sutures were
required to close the opening after its edges were thoroughly
pared. These being introduced transversely, of course the
clamps had to be applied longitudinally, and thus secured.
The edges of the opening came together well enough, but they
were not accurately adapted to each other, owing to *a greater
thickness of one than the other, and the consequent elevation of
the corresponding clamp above its fellow.*

"With this condition of things the patient was put to bed,
and a catheter (English elastic) introduced into the bladder to
convey off as much of the urine as possible. Very little of it,
however, passed through the instrument; it continued its old
course through the vagi-
na. The clamps were al-
lowed to remain the usual
length of time. When I
came to remove them, I
had no need of scissors.
*The whole concern had
sloughed out and lay loose
in the fistulous opening,
now greatly enlarged.*"

Fig. 15 shows the an-
terior wall of the vagina
expanded to the limit in-
dicated by the dilator, and
the different sizes of the
three fistules, together
with their relative posi-
tions .in the different
structures i m p l i c a t e d.
The pair of clamps ap-
plied to the fistule, de-
scribed as located in the
vesico-vaginal septum (a
far more eligible situation
for their use than that of

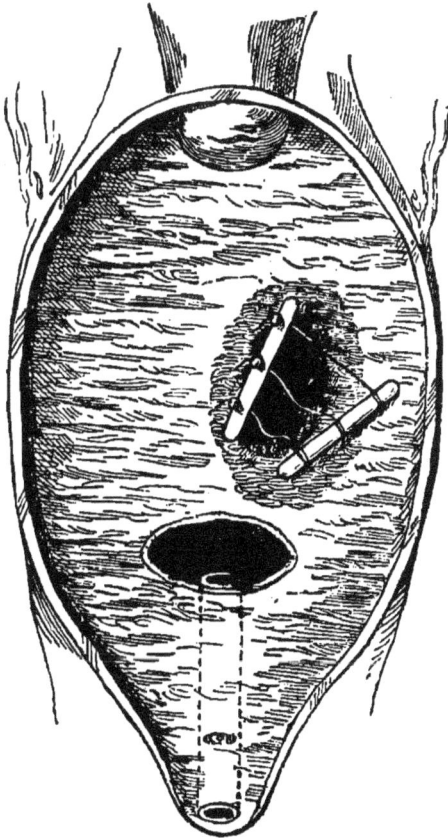

Fig. 15.

either of the other two lesions), are here shown detached entirely from the borders of the fistule, and incrusted with calcareous

deposits from the urine, as found on the twelfth day after the operation. The shaded surfaces around the opening indicate the extent of the ulceration and cutting of the tissues by the apparatus. In addition to all this, there was a general elytritis superinduced by the increased acridity of the urine, arising from the operation and the cutting out of the suture apparatus.

" The result of this operation thoroughly satisfied me that I should never be able to close *successively* the fistulous openings in this case. The whole failure I attributed to the poisonous effect of the urine upon the denuded edges of the fistule, and the raw surfaces caused by the imbedding of the clamps. So well was I convinced of this fact, that I should have discharged the patient without ever making another trial, had not the idea fortunately occurred to me of protection to the approximated edges of one fistule from the irritating effect of the urine passing through the other. From this thought, scarcely need I say, the principle of the *button-suture*—a new application of the interrupted form of suture—originated, and was put into practice.

" Although the principle of protection was suggested in the combinations above stated, by the peculiarity of this case, yet the first trial of it was not made here."

The patient, after this operation, returned home to recuperate her health, and was not regularly treated again for about eighteen months. The case will be referred to again, and the final result stated, in the class of urethro-vesico-vaginal fistules, to be considered farther on.

Suffice it to say, it was not until after I had performed two other operations with the clamp-suture, in two different cases (the first successfully in a vesico-utero-vaginal fistule, and the second unsuccessfully in a vesico-vaginal fistule), that the principle of this new form of suture, which I accidentally discovered in the process of buttoning my vest, came to be applied. The first trial of it was made after this same second operation, it being a third failure with the clamp-suture in the case. Consequently, the introduction of the case, or rather the conclusion of its history, since it has al-

ready been related in part (Case IX of the series, Julia Mc-
Duffie), properly belongs here. To this will be added three
other cases, two not belonging to the series (they never having been operated upon with the clamp-suture), and one, Case
VIII of the series, Delia, previously operated upon unsuccessfully by Dr. Sims.

The object I had in view in presenting at such length the
foregoing history and treatment of Matilda Stamper was to
show that, after adopting my modification of Dr. Sims's form
of the lever-speculum, my supported knee-chest position, and,
finally, my system of gradual preparatory treatment, all important principles with which to extend the usefulness of the
clamp-suture, but which, in this case, utterly failed in their
object, on account of the defectiveness of this form of suture,
there was a sequence of incidents, from first to last, important to note, as showing the pressing necessity, at this juncture, of the invention of the button interrupted suture. By
its adoption and successful application in the cases of Julia
McDuffie and Kitty Johnston, the two first cases in which it
was employed, not only was the great value of these general
principles demonstrated conclusively, but the philosophy of
the suture itself was put to the severest test as to the range
of its usefulness, which it would be difficult to overestimate,
even at the present time.

The sequence of the several improved stages of treatment
thus far discussed, and the dates of their adoption, may be
summed up as follows:

1. The modification of Dr. Sims's form of the lever-
speculum, in June, 1853.

2. The utilization of the supported knee-chest position, in
the spring of 1854.

3. The adoption and first successful application of the
principle of gradual preparatory treatment for cicatricial contractions of the vagina as complications of vesico-vaginal fistules, in February, 1855.

4. The invention and first employment of the button
interrupted suture, embodying the new principle of shield-

ing the denuded edges of the fistule from all extraneous influences, and of a special mode of adjusting all interrupted metallic sutures in the vagina without the intervention of the fingers, May 12, 1855.

5. The utilization of the uterus, by pulling it down and making it subservient, without incisions, to the reparation of all fistules attended with loss of tissue, August 23, 1855.

The following are extracts taken from the published reports of the four cases above referred to, presenting seven fistules in two classes, five vesico-vaginal and one vesico-utero vaginal (two of them presenting grave complications), and all closed by the *button-suture procedure* at seven operations:

A.—Vesico-vaginal Fistule—Small Size—Situation in the Septum near Cervix Uteri and Left Lateral Wall of Vagina —Cicatricial Hardness and Thickness of Left Border of Fistule—Distortion of Vaginal Tract at Same Point—Three Operations with Clamp-Suture unsuccessful—Used jointly in Third Operation Bozeman's Improved Lever-Speculum, and his Supported Knee-Chest Position for Anesthesia—Good Exposure of Fistule—Result: Total Failure as in the Two Preceding Operations—Inapplicability of Clamp-Suture to such an Abnormal State of the Structures proved—Some Two Weeks afterward Button Interrupted Suture invented—Applied now for the First Time under precisely the Same Circumstances as attended the Third Operation with Clamp-Suture—Result: Complete Cure without the Slightest Irritation of the Structures involved—Invention of Suture Adjuster and Demonstration of its Practical Utility at Same Time—This Instrument Indispensable for the Successful Use of all Wire Sutures in the Vagina without the Intervention of the Fingers—Applicability of the New Procedure to such an Abnormal State of the Structures proved beyond Question.

Julia McDuffie, colored, aged twenty-one, readmitted for treatment April 12, 1855. It will be recollected that this case first came under the joint care of Dr. Sims and myself for treatment in Montgomery, Ala., early in March, 1853. It was then stated that Dr. Sims operated upon the case with his clamp-suture (see Fig. 9), which proved a total failure from ulceration and the cutting out of the clamp on the left side, this border of the fistule being thickened and indurated ; and that I repeated the same operation, under the same circumstances, about two months and a half later, June 1, 1853, with the same unfortunate result. It will be recollected that it was the cicatricial contraction of the vagina in the case which led me at that time to make a modification of Dr. Sims's form of the lever-speculum with regard to the length and shape of the blade, and the angle formed by this with the handle of the instrument, as shown in Fig. 11.

Below is the concluding part of the history of the case,[1] and it will here be seen in my report that I avoided direct reference to Dr. Sim's failure with his clamp-suture :

"The following spring [March 15, 1853] she was *operated upon according to the method of Dr. Sims, but was not relieved.* She came under my charge a short time afterward, and, upon examination, I readily discovered a circular opening of about the size of a No. 6 catheter, occupying the vesico-vaginal septum near the neck of the uterus and a little to the left side. On the right side the tissues were in a normal condition, but on the left very much indurated. After due preparation of the system, I applied the clamp-suture in the usual way. On the thirteenth day I examined and found that the clamp on the left side had cut entirely out, and the aperture considerably enlarged.

"Shortly after this unsuccessful operation the patient's general health became very much impaired, and it was thought advisable to allow her to return home. I heard no more of the case until April 12, 1855, when she was again placed under my care, having, in the mean time, entirely regained her usual good health. I found, on making an examination, that the fistule was somewhat smaller than when I last saw her, but the induration of the left border still existed. Aside from this latter circumstance, I considered the case altogether favorable, and felt very confident that an operation would prove successful. Accordingly, on the 17th of April, I applied the clamp-

[1] See Case I, *op. cit.*

suture again. The edges of .the fistule came together beautifully, but, owing to the *indurated condition on the left side, the corresponding clamp could not be made to imbed itself, and consequently rested on a plane higher than the one on the opposite side.* Notwithstanding this rather unfavorable feature, I was very sanguine of success.

"On the thirteenth day I examined the parts, and, to my great mortification, saw that the left clamp had again cut out, and thus enlarged the opening." (See Fig. 16.) This was my last operation with the clamp-suture.

"After two (three in all) such signal failures with the only operation that I then considered worthy of confidence, I was much discouraged, and had serious thoughts of abandoning the case altogether ; but it was only a week or two subsequently that the principle of the button-suture first suggested itself to me, and I immediately determined to subject the case to an experimental trial. All things being ready, on the 12th of May (1855), I put the new method in operation.

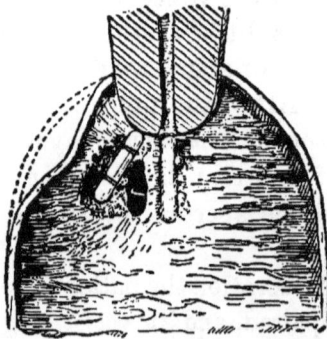
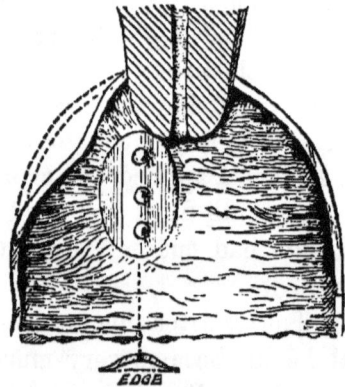

Fig. 16.   Fig. 17.

"Everything seemed to progress favorably. On the thirteenth day I removed the apparatus, and, to my great delight, found the fistule completely closed, and not the slightest evidence of irritation except what might be naturally expected around each suture."

Fig. 17 shows the operation completed, and the adaptation of the apparatus to the parts, the general condition of the latter being precisely the same as in the previous three operations, with the increase added each time, of course, of the cicatricial hardness of the tissues, arising from the ulceration and cutting out of the clamps, which had to be placed on the thickened border of the fistule.

In the construction of this button-suture, the silver wire and perforated shot used were, of course, borrowed from the now discarded clamp-suture method of Dr. Sims; but it is proper to state in this connection that Dr. Henry S. Levert,[1] of Mobile, Ala., was the first, certainly in this country, to point out the innoxiousness of silver wire, and its superiority on that account to ligatures made of organic substances. Dr. J. P. Mettauer, of Prince Edward, Va., three years later demonstrated the advantages of simple interrupted lead sutures, secured by twisting over those silk for recto-vaginal fistule and laceration of the perineum. My form of suture was, properly speaking, a button interrupted suture, being, in principle of action, a combination and extension of the old principles of the interrupted and twisted sutures. The originality, therefore, was in the combination and extension of these two principles, just as the clamp-suture of Dr. Sims was a combination and extension of the old principles of the interrupted and quill sutures; his originality being the substitution of Levert's silver wire for silk, and of small, round perforated lead bars for the quills, and in the use of perforated shot to secure the whole.

As an essential feature of the radical change of principle and form of suture made at this juncture in the history of the subject, I deem it important to introduce, in connection with the same, the accompanying illustration of my suture adjuster (Fig. 18), as a means of quick coaptation of the denuded edges of the fistule without the intervention of the fingers inside the vagina. This consisted in doubling or shouldering large-size silver sutures, one after another, and thus quickly drawing the denuded edges of the fistule in close and firm contact; the loops in the wire in all cases being

[1] *American Journal of the Medical Sciences*, May, 1829.

sufficient to hold the parts together until the process was completed, and the line of closure could be examined, as shown by Fig. 19. When the latter was found unsatisfactory, from defective or ragged paring, it was easy to undo the loops and complete properly this important step of the operation,

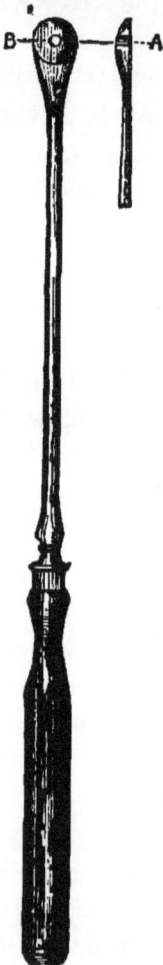

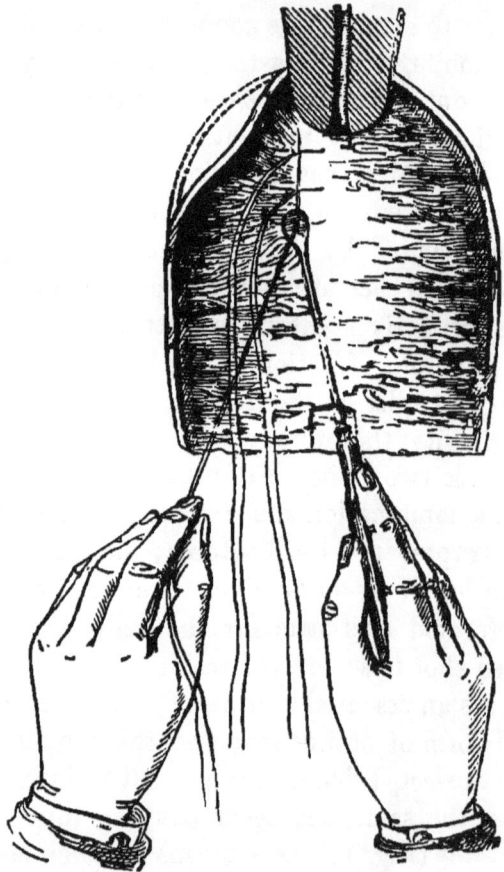

Fig. 18.   Fig. 19.

thus making it mathematically accurate. The coaptation of the denuded edges being now finished, and the line of union seen to be perfect, the next step was to hermetically seal it, by sliding down upon the doubled and shouldered wires the perforated button or shield over the structures and then firmly securing it. This was effected with perforated shot slid down upon the wires in a similar way, and compressed with a pair of strong forceps successively upon the top of the button, thus completing the procedure in two distinct stages.

No such instrument for specially adjusting wire sutures had been used prior to this date. Surgeons[1] formerly had been in the habit of putting together the two ends of each wire outside the vagina, and then twisting them like a cord from right to left, or left to right; thus the two edges of the denuded fistule were slowly dragged into contact and loosely or firmly coaptated as the chance experience of the operator might determine. In the operation with the clamp-suture,[2] such an instrument was not required, as both ends of each of the several wires had to be disposed of and secured separately.

Whether, in the use of this suture adjuster, the two ends of the several wires be first passed through the hole outside the vulva, and the instrument then be slid down upon them to the extent of forming a small, closed loop and coaptating the edges of the fistule, as preparatory to their fixation with the button and perforated shot; or whether the hole in it be slit out to its extremity and the two ends of the several wires be received into it inside the vagina, where the instrument is firmly held against the edges of the fistule, preparatory to their fixation by twisting alone, as in the use of simple interrupted sutures—is a matter of no consequence ; the principle is one and the same. The instrument may be called a *suture adjuster*, or, as variously modified, a "fulcrum," a "prop," a "support," or anything else; but the *originality and priority* of its use constitute a part of the invention and first employment of the button-suture, May 12, 1855.

The Woman's Hospital of the State of New York threw its doors open on May 1, 1855. My last operation with the clamp-suture, as above shown, was performed thirteen days

[1] Mettauer, *loc. cit.*, 1832 ; Gosset, *Lancet*, November 21, 1834.
[2] Sims, *American Journal of the Medical Sciences*, January, 1852.

before, and my first with the procedure of the button-interrupted suture twelve days after that date. While all this was going on, Dr. Sims, the surgeon-in-chief of that institution, was just about beginning the second series of cases with his clamp-suture, to be hereafter presented. In that connection I shall show the extraordinary coincidence that *his* last operation with the clamp-suture took place in the Woman's Hopital, in the case of Emily Stebbins, on May 12, 1856, twelve days after the first account of my new procedure appeared in print.[1] I shall also show, in this connection, that Dr. Sims performed, in the same institution, his first operation with the simple-interrupted suture secured by twisting (as first practiced by Mettauer with lead sutures) in the case of Ellen Quidre, about six weeks later, June 23, 1856;[2] and that, in this new procedure of his, the modifications of my suture-adjuster, Fig. 18, under the name of "fulcrum of support," and of my sponge-dilator, Fig. 13, under the designation of "glass plug," form distinguishing features without which even the most skillful operator at the present time would be almost as powerless as he was with his old clamp-suture in endeavoring to master the real difficulties appertaining to the treatment of the simple class of vesico-vaginal fistules.

B.—*Two Fistules, one Vesico-vaginal and one Vesico-uterovaginal—Situation of Former below Center of Septum and of Latter in Bas-fond of Bladder, against Cervix Uteri— Between the two Openings, Cicatricial Contraction of Vaginal Tract down to the Size of a Surgeon's Probe—Urine exceedingly acrid and loaded with Triple Phosphates—Vaginitis of High Grade—Extensive Excoriations of the Labia Majora, Buttocks, and Thighs—All Five of the Principles embodied in the Button-Suture Procedure beautifully illustrated—Closure of the Vesico-vaginal Fistule at One Operation; Denuded Edges of Fistule effectually shielded from all Extraneous Influences —Cicatricial Contraction of Vagina attacked and overcome*

[1] *Louisville Review*, May 1, 1856.
[2] "Silver Sutures in Surgery," 1858.

—*Anterior Lip of Cervix Uteri without Incisions made sub-servient to Closure of the Vesico-utero-vaginal Fistule at One Operation—First Step toward superseding the Necessity of cutting loose the Cervix Uteri from the Bladder to avoid Traction upon the Sutures, as previously recommended by Jobert de Lamballe—Patient discharged cured.*

Kitty Johnston,[1] colored, aged eighteen, applied for treatment May 24, 1855, under the following circumstances : "Found the thighs, the buttocks, and the labia majora almost completely incrusted by calcareous matter, and so sensitive that the least effort to separate them caused excruciating pain. Before the vagina could be explored, this deposit had to be removed, and even then the suffering was considerable, owing to an extremely irritable condition of the organ, and a protrusion of the mucous coat of the bladder through the fistulous opening. When the speculum was introduced, *the posterior wall of the vagina could not be raised up with the usual facility. This I soon found resulted from a morbid attachment of its two walls. The adhesion extended obliquely across from the right side of the cervix uteri to the left side of the vagina, thus concealing from view the os uteri, and rendering an exploration of the entire canal impossible.* A fistulous opening [vesico-vaginal] three quarters of an inch in length occupied the vesico-vaginal septum, and extended from near the beginning of the urethra obliquely upward and to the left, terminating abruptly at the point of contraction. Here a careful examination revealed a small opening which allowed a probe to pass into the *cul-de-sac* above, and from thence into the bladder, showing clearly that another fistule [vesico-utero-vaginal] existed in this situation. [See Fig. 20.]

"Having thus ascertained the true condition of things, I became satisfied that two operations would be required. The fistule first described was accessible, and demanded my first attention, owing to its larger size and the very irritable state of the mucous coat of the bladder which protruded through it. I thought it advisable, however, before attempting any operation, to improve the patient's general health.

. . . .

---
[1] Case II, *op. cit.*

"*June 12.*—[The patient being in the supported knee-chest position] I proceeded to apply the button-suture to the lower opening. Much difficulty was encountered in paring the edges, owing to the great resistance of the patient and the herniated

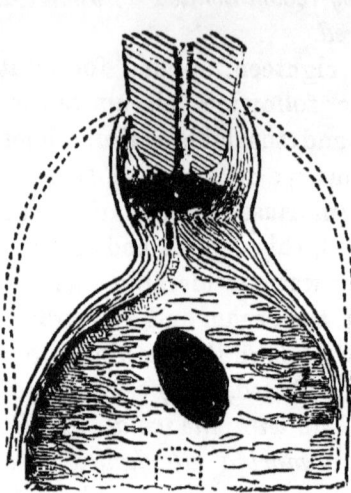

Fig. 20.

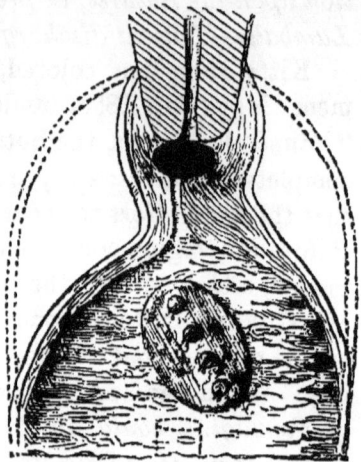

Fig. 21.

condition of the mucous coat of the bladder. Four sutures were required; the button was seven eighths of an inch in length, and about five eighths in width. [See Fig. 21.]

"For two or three days after the operation there was considerable fever and pain in the hypogastric region, and I feared something serious might result; but things soon took a favorable turn, and the case seemed to do well until about the seventh day. At this time a great discharge of urine occurred from the vagina, and my first impression was that the sutures had given way; but, upon examining the parts carefully, I discovered the whole of the difficulty to depend upon tympanitic distention of the bowels, attended at times with powerful peristaltic action. . . .

"Feeling a little uneasiness as to the result, notwithstanding the discovery of the source of the trouble, I determined on the ninth day to remove the apparatus. Upon the introduction of the speculum into the vagina, the parts presented a most unpromising appearance; the mucous membrane was of a deep-red color, and the button completely incrusted with earthy matter. I now had a firm presentiment that all was not right ; but when the sutures were clipped and the button raised, I found to my great satisfaction that union of the parts was perfect.

"In a few weeks I made preparation for the other operation by *breaking up the morbid adhesion between the two walls of the vagina, so as to expose the fistulous opening above. To prevent reunion of the parts, a bag made of oil-silk and stuffed with bits of sponge was introduced into the vagina. This was renewed daily, and injections of cold water used, by which means the upper extremity of the vagina was dilated in a few weeks to its normal size and the fistule well exposed.*

"*August 23.*—Everything appearing as favorable as could be expected, I proceeded to operate. Only three sutures were required ; but, as in the former operation, I had much diffi-culty, owing to the resistance of the patient. Tympanites supervened again several days after the operation, and caused the patient a good deal of suf-fering ; but with this exception the case did well. [Fig. 22 shows the vagina restored to its normal caliber, the form of su-ture used, and the utilization of the anterior lip of the cervix uteri for closing the fistule without incisions or dissection of the cervix uteri from the bladder, as insisted upon by

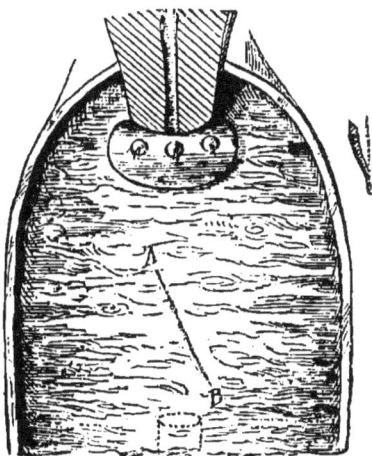

Fig. 22.

Jobert de Lamballe. *A B* is the line of cicatrization of the first fistule closed.]

"On the ninth day [September 1, 1855] I removed the ap-paratus, and had the satisfaction of finding an entirely success-ful result; not the slightest irritation had been produced. The improvement of the patient in every respect was very rapid, and when I discharged her in September she was as active and sprightly as though she had never had a sick day.

"*Remarks.*—The bad health of the patient, the existence of two fistulous openings, a herniated condition of the mucous coat of the bladder, *a morbid attachment of the two walls of the vagina, and an exceedingly irritating quality of the urine, were all circumstances which strongly militated against the treatment. It is, indeed, one of the most remarkable cases that have ever come under my observation, and I may add that a better case for illustrating some of the advantages claimed for the button-suture, and especially that of protection to the denuded edges of the fistule from the poisonous effects of the urine, could not have been selected. After removing the button employed in the first operation, its very shape and size were found impressed upon the parts over which it rested during the healing process, and the pale-red color of the mucous membrane contrasted beautifully with the deep-red and fiery appearance of that which had been exposed to the urine escaping through the upper opening.*"

C.—*Two Vesico-vaginal Fistules, one situated at Center of Septum, and the other near Cervix Uteri—Latter not discovered until after the Former was closed—No Complications present—Each Fistule closed at a Single Operation by the Button-Suture Procedure—Patient discharged cured.*

Dinah,[1] a colored woman, aged forty-seven years, applied for treatment, June 28, 1855 :

" Upon examination, I found a fistule near the center of the vesico-vaginal septum, circular in shape, and sufficiently large to admit the index-finger into the bladder. Supposing this to be the only opening, on the 5th day of July I applied the button-suture. On the tenth day it was removed, and the parts found to be perfectly united, not the slightest irritation having been produced by the apparatus. In a few days afterward the patient was allowed to get up ; but, to my surprise, there was still dribbling of urine. I apprehended, therefore, that the newly formed cicatrix had given way, and there was a reproduction of the fistule ; but, on making an examination, I discovered that such was not the case. I was now at a loss to account for the appearance of urine ; but, upon a more careful exploration of the vagina, I found another very small opening, situated far up on the right side, at least an inch from the one I had closed.

[1] Case III, *op. cit.*

"The whole difficulty was now explained. Another operation was required ; but, owing to the bad health of the patient, I was not able to perform it until the 10th of September.

"The fistule, although small, had a peculiarity I had never met with before. It was valvulous—i. e., the opening through the vaginal part of the septum did not correspond to that of the vesical. Two sutures were sufficient to bring the edges together. Things went on well, and on the tenth day I removed the apparatus, and found union perfect.

"*Remarks.*—In this instance the fistulous openings were of eighteen years' standing, the patient old, and her general health not very good ; yet the result was as prompt and decided as could have been desired. *One of the great advantages claimed for the button-suture—namely, protection to the denuded edges of the fistule—was again forcibly illustrated in this case.*"

D.—*Two Vesico-vaginal Fistules—Situation below Center of Septum on a Transverse Line, one to the Left of Median Line, and the other reaching to the Right Lateral Wall of Vagina—Both Angular Fistules, resulting from Closure in the Middle of a Large Opening after Ten or more Operations with the Clamp-Suture in the Hands of Dr. Sims—No Complications present, further than the Co-existence of Two Fistules and the Cicatricial Hardening of the Tissues, resulting from the Repeated Cutting-out of the Clamps—Each Fistule closed at One Operation by the Button-Suture Procedure—Patient discharged cured.*

Delia,[1] a mulatto girl, aged twenty-five years, servant of Dr. Sims, was re-admitted for further treatment September 10, 1855. The case, it will be recollected, was treated jointly by Dr. Sims and myself in May, 1853. He performed his last operation with the clamp-suture at that time, the after-treatment being conducted by me. He used a pair of clamps upon each fistule at the same sitting. Nothing unusual attended the after-treatment. When I examined the parts, however, on the twelfth day, I found that both upper clamps had ulcerated out, and the result was a total failure. It will also be recollected that the case had then been under treatment between three and four years, and that Dr. Sims had, from first to last, performed

---

[1] Case IV, *op. cit.*

ten or more operations with the clamp-suture. Here is the patient's own brief account of her previous history, to which are appended the results of my examination and of my operations with the button-suture at this juncture. In my first report it will again be seen that I avoided direct reference to the number of failures with the clamp-suture by Dr. Sims:

. "She also states that she was sent to New Orleans, and there treated [after confinement in 1846] for a long time, with but little, if any, benefit. *Since then she has been operated upon several times according to the method of Dr. Sims, but the relief afforded was only partial.*

"Upon examination, I found two fistulous openings—one about two inches from the cervix (uteri), and a little to the left side; the other, a little larger, was situated far to the right, at a point just where the anterior and posterior walls of

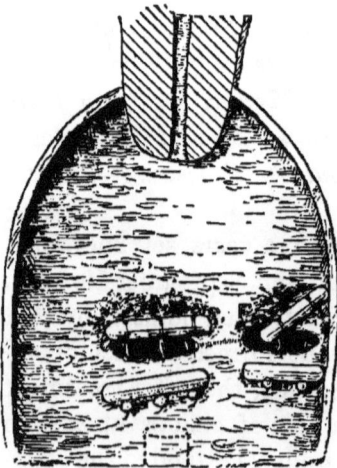

Fig. 23.

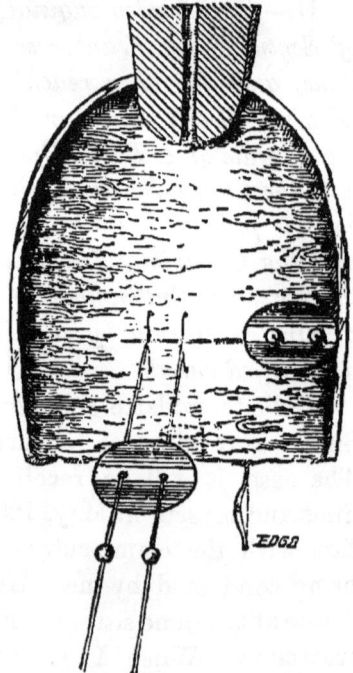

Fig. 24.

the vagina become continuous. [Fig. 23 shows the situation of the two fistules, and the partially detached clamp-suture upon each, as I found them on the twelfth day after Dr. Sims's last operation, May 20, 1853. The dark line between the two fistules indicates the cicatrix of the closure of the fistule in the middle by Dr. Sims in his previous operations.]

"On the 10th of September [1855], I proceeded to apply the button-suture to the larger opening. It was my intention to close the other also at the same time, but the patient preferred to wait. Only two sutures were required, and on the tenth day I removed the apparatus, and found union perfect.

"October the 18th, I operated upon the other fistule. This I found presented *the same peculiarity that was observed in the preceding case, in being of a valvular form.* Only two sutures were required, and on the tenth day I removed the apparatus, and found adhesion perfect, without the slightest irritation in the surrounding parts.

[Fig. 24 shows the situation of the two fistules to be the same as in Fig. 23, the one on the right illustrating the button in position, as it appeared at the time of removal; and the other on the left showing the button ready to be slid down upon the sutures and secured with the perforated shot following it, which resulted in a complete cure, October 28, 1855.]

"*Remarks.*—The result in this case was as satisfactory as could be desired; it needs no comments. If it proves anything, it is that the button-suture was better adapted to the case than the clamp-suture, which latter had been long and perseveringly tried.

"CONCLUSIONS.—Having now finished a description of my mode of treating vesico-vaginal fistule, together with the narration of all the cases in which it has been employed, I propose, in conclusion, to compare its results with those obtained by other methods.

"Since the 12th of May last [1855], I have performed seven successive operations without a single failure. This is the amount of my experience with the button-suture. Now, to form anything like a proper estimate of the several modes of treatment heretofore recommended, it is necessary first to ascertain what proportion of the operations, according to each, have been successful when compared with the whole number performed. In this way only can their respective merits be properly set forth. To effect this object I have examined, so far as my opportunities allowed, the records, both of Europe and this country; but, as the data are imperfect, I have not been able to arrive at very satisfactory conclusions.

"Chelius speaks of Wutzer as having had the greatest success. Of eighteen cases operated upon, three were radically cured. We are not informed how many operations were performed in all.

"Jobert, by the anaplastic process, cures, I am induced to believe, about one half of his cases. What proportion of his operations fail, I have not been able to learn.

"Mr. Henry Earle is said to have operated thirty times upon one case before succeeding. The failures here were as twenty-nine to one.

"Mr. Brown operated ten times upon three cases, and obtained one successful result. The failures here were as nine to one.

"Dr. Hayward operated twenty times upon nine cases, and obtained three successful results. The failures here were as seventeen to three.

"I am not prepared to state positively what proportion of the whole number of operations performed, according to the method of Dr. Sims, has been successful. Judging from my own experience, and from what I have seen of it in the practice of others [referring alone to that of Dr. Sims], I am inclined to think that the average is not over one half.[1]

---

[1] "A few weeks since there appeared in the ' *New York Medical Gazette* ' a notice of the number of the ' *Louisville Review* ' containing the above article, in which the writer says that I am mistaken in regard to Dr. Sims's success, and asserts that he (Dr. Sims) has cured, during his residence in New York, thirty cases without a failure.

"From this it would seem that I had done Dr. Sims great injustice. While I here disclaim any such intention, I will simply add that my language in reference to his and other operations, as compared with mine, is explicit, and I am surprised it should have been construed into a meaning so unjust.

"That Dr. Sims has done what is claimed for him [with his clamp-suture], I have not the slightest doubt; but this fact has no bearing upon the statement made by me. The point which I endeavored to arrive at was, what proportion of the number of operations performed according to each of the different methods indicated had been successful. The opinion expressed as to the *clamp-*

"In regard to my own cases, it may be supposed by some that they were all peculiarly favorable, which accounts for my unprecedented success; but this was not the case. A reference to their individual histories will show that they were quite the reverse. The very fact of two of them having resisted the repeated application of the clamp-suture [in Dr. Sims's own hands], is proof sufficient upon this point. The other two were each double fistules, and therefore very unfavorable. One of them, Case II, I consider the most un-promising I have ever seen that was at all curable.

"In conclusion, I freely acknowledge that the results thus far obtained by the use of the button-suture, although so remarkably successful, do not amount to a sufficient num-ber to justify an indisputable claim to its superiority over all other procedures; and I do not, therefore, urge its adoption by the profession without further trial. This is all I ask for it at present. My limited experience with it has led me to believe that the principles upon which it acts are more nearly correct than any heretofore suggested; but if, upon more careful examination, this be found not true, it will simply prove that the success of my seven operations was a most re-markable and heretofore unheard-of coincidence.[1]

"MONTGOMERY, *Jan. 1, 1856.*"

suture was principally based upon my own experience with it. This amounted to eight operations, six of which had been complete failures. If I am in error as to the average success of other operators with it, it remains to be determined by statistical facts, which are not before me, and, so far as my knowledge ex-tends, have never been published.

"As additional support to the advantages claimed for the button-suture in my paper, I will state that, since it was prepared for the press, I have per-formed eight more operations, making in all fifteen. My twelfth operation was a partial failure. All of the others were entirely successful.

"*July, 1856.*"

[1] I would remark, in this connection, that the statement of the writer in the "*New York Medical Gazette,*" as set forth in the foregoing foot-note, was purely gratuitous, as I have since satisfied myself from a careful examination of the subject. Dr. Sims had not then cured thirty cases of vesico-vaginal fistule with his clamp-suture. His cures at that date, including all before and after coming to New York, within a period of about eleven years, exceeded very little, if at all, half the number stated, as I shall show in this study of the subject farther on.

SIMPLE STATEMENT OF THE PRECEDING FOUR CASES TREATED
BY THE BUTTON-SUTURE PROCEDURE BETWEEN MAY 12
AND OCTOBER 18, 1855.

Classification.—Of seven fistules in four cases, there
were of the first class six vesico-vaginal fistules, two single,
two double, four simple, and two complicated. Of the complicated ones, the first presented induration and thickening
of left border of the fistule, with cicatricial contraction and
distortion of the corresponding lateral wall of the vagina
opposite the same point; while the second combined the co-
existence of a vesico-utero-vaginal fistule with almost complete occlusion of the vagina below, general vaginitis of a
high grade, alkaline urine, calcareous deposits, internal and
external excoriations, etc.

The vesico-utero-vaginal fistule, belonging to the second
class, was attended with loss of tissue and the co-existence of
a vesico-vaginal fistule, this being the complicated case with
partial occlusion, etc., described in the preceding class.

Number of Operations.—Upon seven fistules in two
classes, seven operations were performed. Six vesico-vaginal
fistules got six direct operations. One vesico-utero-vaginal
fistule got one direct operation.

General Results.—The treatment of seven fistules of all
classes yielded these results: Seven fistules were all completely closed—100 per cent.

Special Results.—Of seven fistules treated in different
classes, six vesico-vaginal fistules of the first class were all
completely closed—100 per cent; one vesico-utero-vaginal
fistule of the second class was completely closed—100 per
cent.

Average number of operations—one to each fistule closed.

Previous Operations with the Clamp-Suture.—Eleven by
Sims, in Cases A and D—all failures. Two by Bozeman, in
Case A—both failures.

Of thirteen operations in all with the clamp-suture, performed by both surgeons, three were upon one small vesico-
vaginal fistule, complicated with induration and thickening

of one border of the opening, with cicatricial contraction and distortion of the vaginal tract in the same situation, and ten were upon one vesico-vaginal fistule of medium size, without complications, which resulted in closure in the middle, leaving two angular openings as the final resulting failure.

This brings us back again to the line of continuous narration of the remaining seven cases of the class of vesico-vaginal fistules.[1]

---

[1] It will not be irrelevant to here state, *en passant*, that of the twenty remaining cases of this series, only three were ever cured with the clamp-suture—one of the class of urethro-vesico-vaginal fistule, by Dr. R. D. Mussey, of Cincinnati, attended with slight loss of tissue, as illustrated by Fig. 4, and two of the class of vesico-utero-vaginal fistule, by myself, unattended with loss of tissue: the laceration in one extending into the anterior lip of the cervix uteri in this form, ⋀, and, in the other, simply up to the anterior lip, as illustrated by Fig. 5.